W9-BMY-156

WILDLIFE HOSPITAL

Stories From The
Northwoods Wildlife Center

by

Sybil B. Ferguson

Photographs by

BOB BALDWIN

Copyright Information - *Wildlife Hospital*

© 1991 Sybil Ferguson

Published by NorthWord Press, Inc.
Box 1360
Minocqua, WI 54548

ISBN 1-55971-072-1

For a free catalog describing NorthWord's line of
nature books and gifts, call 1-800-336-5666.

All photographs contained herein copyright
© Robert W. Baldwin, and may not
be reproduced in any form without
express permission of the photographer.

WILDLIFE HOSPITAL

by
Sybil Ferguson

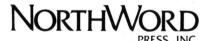

PRESS, INC

P.O. Box 1360
Minocqua, Wisconsin 54548

CONTENTS

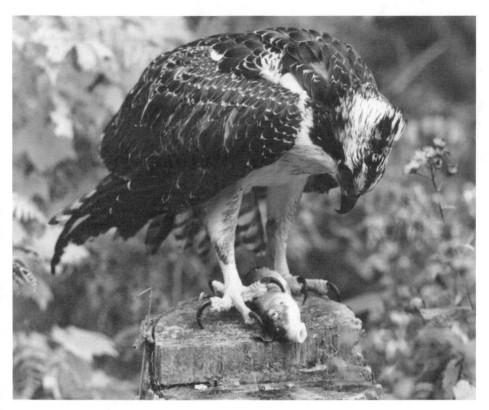

A juvenile osprey about to dine on a big sucker.

"For the animal shall not be measured by man. In a world older and more complete than ours they move finished and complete, gifted with extensions of the senses we have lost or never attained, living by voices we shall never hear. They are not brethren, they are not underlings; they are other nations, caught with ourselves in the net of life and time, fellow prisoners of the splendor and travail of the earth."

-Henry Beston

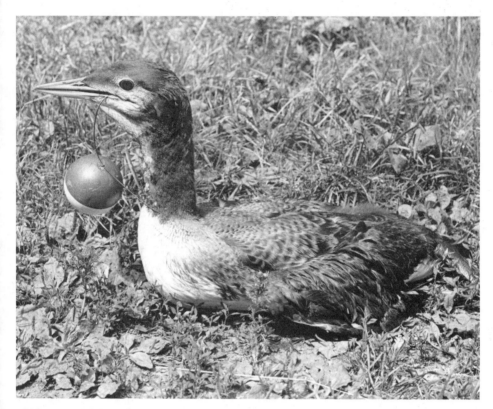

This immature loon that has swallowed a fish hook is typical of the kind of patient that comes to the Northwoods Wildlife Center for treatment and rehabilitation.

AUTHOR'S NOTE

All of these stories are true in essence, but in some the details have been added to fill them out. We know, for instance, that a screech owl was transferred from South Dakota where it was a tourist attraction in a gas station. We know that a barred owl was raised by a woman in Ashland, WI. We know that our golden eagle was shot in Wyoming, probably by a sheep rancher who wanted to protect his lambs. These basic truths have been turned into stories of what might have happened. When we know the facts, they are told exactly as they happened. As you read, you will know the difference. Have fun! It was fun to write!

INTRODUCTION

Those of you who are familiar with **Dr. Wildlife** and **I Never Met An Animal I Didn't Like** will remember Rory Foster and his wildlife hospital. If you haven't read Rory's books, I suggest that you do. They are a good read. You may be wondering why he is not writing the third book, and why I am. I am sorry to have to tell you that Dr. Rory Foster died on September 24, 1987 at the age of 37 of Amyotrophic Lateral Sclerosis, a progressive paralysis for which there is presently no known cure.

But in his short lifetime, Rory Foster made a difference, which is all any of us aspire to in a longer lifetime. For purposes of this book, his prime achievement was the founding of a hospital and rehabilitation center for injured, ill, and orphaned wild animals. This hospital was incorporated as a separate entity in 1979; eleven years prior to this writing. Enough money was raised to build a hospital building next to the Foster Smith Animal Hospital, and the Center opened on the 19th of June in 1982. Rory's first book is the story of how the hospital came into being. (No, the mortgage isn't paid off, yet!)

In 1982, when the new building opened, the executive director and licensed rehabilitator was Mark Blackbourn, the only employee. All the rest of the staff was composed of volunteers, this writer among them.

You will read very little about Rory Foster in this book. You will read about Mark; about Dave, the disabled Vietnam vet who volunteered in 1982 and is still there; about Bill, the director who followed Mark; about Tony, who managed the Center between Bill and Warren; and you will learn about Warren, the present executive director and Jacqueline Quesnell, the center's rehabilitator. And you will get to know me, too.

You will meet Orson, the great horned owl, Bart, the barred owl, and Clawdia, the bald eagle. You will read about loons and raccoons, babies of all species, our successes and our failures (we can't win 'em all). And I hope, like Rory's books, this one turns out to be a "good read."

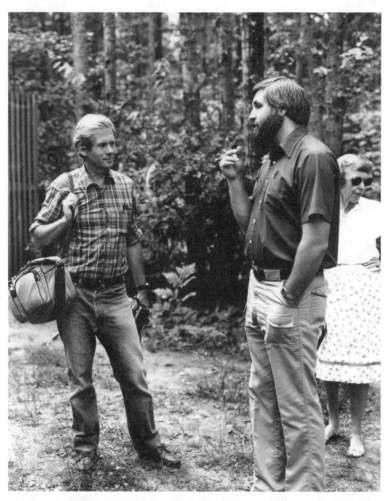

World-famous wildlife artist Robert Bateman frequently ventures down from his native Canada to visit the Center to sketch, make field notes and photograph its residents. Here, he visits with Mark Blackbourn.

PART I:
SOME OF
OUR PATIENTS

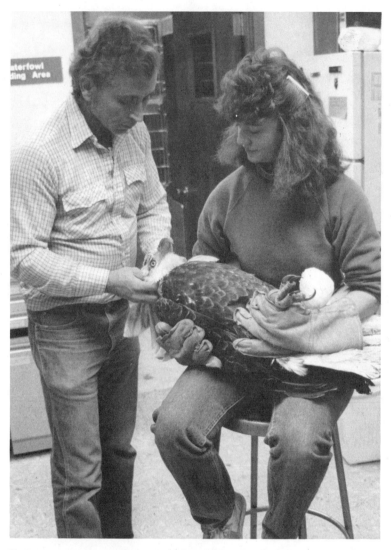

Dave examines a trap-injured bald eagle that is being held by Kris Doss, a summer intern. Injured raptor talons are dressed with "ball" bandages so the talon can wrap around a ball of gauze and need not be flattened out.

THE EAGLES
HAVE LANDED

"I never meant for this to happen!" The big man with a big box shoved his way through the door and into the front hall. "As God is my witness, I never meant for this to happen. I been trapping all my life, since I was a kid, and this is the worst thing that ever happened." His eyes were misty, and his throat was tight.

Mark set the box down and opened the flaps cautiously. "Oh, my God!" he breathed, and went to the back for the heavy welder's gloves he uses to handle the animals. The trapper took out his blue bandanna and with a mighty sniff wiped his entire face roughly.

Mark returned and opened the box again. Two fierce eyes glared at him. Mark carefully placed his hands on the big bird's shoulders to control its wings and lifted it out of the box. "An eagle," he said softly. "A bald eagle."

"It's never happened to me before," the trapper repeated. "and never will again. I'm pulling my traps soon as I get home. And I'll bury them," he added loudly, "So's nobody else can use them."

While he was talking, Mark cradled the magnificent bird on its back in his arms, as if he were holding a baby. This exposed the eagle's talons. Both were mashed and bloody. One foot hung by a flap of skin, the bone severed completely. The other was missing two toes. Mark stood silently holding the doomed eagle.

The intricate system of nerve and muscle and tendon that activates an eagle's talons had been destroyed beyond repair. Possibly the feet could be healed, but the bird would never hunt again, and would never be able to perch. Despite the fact that the rest of the bird was whole and healthy, it would probably have to be euthanized. Misery settled like a cloud on the Wildlife Center.

The trapper filled out the admission form and left, head down. Still holding the eagle, Mark said, "Go get Marty." I hurried down the hall to the vet hospital, but had to wait. Marty was seeing a patient. I was very much aware of the bleeding eagle, and when Marty stuck his head out of the exam room door to ask for something from his assistants, I grabbed him and told him what had happened. "Be there," promised Marty, and disappeared back into the room.

There was nothing to do but wait. Mark had taken the eagle into the treatment room just as Dave came in the back door from feeding outside animals. Together, they cleaned the feet gently. If Marty could do anything, they were ready.

Marty hurried in. He swore as he saw the injury. After a close and careful examination, he said, "Dead bird."

Mark nodded. "I thought so."

"I can sew him up, but even with micro-surgery, you can't ever be sure the talons would work. X-ray him. Stabilize him, and we'll get him ready for the Raptor Center." Marty went back to his dogs and cats.

The Raptor Center, at the University of Minnesota College of Veterinary Medicine, specializes in treating birds of prey. All injured and ill eagles from the state of Wisconsin are transported there for treatment. If anything could be done for our eagle, they could do it. Mark called the director, Pat Redig, and told him the eagle would be coming, that the time of arrival depended upon the condition of the bird, and when it would be safe to transfer him. Next it was necessary to alert the airline that an eagle would be "flying" to the Raptor Center. Airlines all over the country transport eagles free of charge so long as they know ahead of time, and the bird is in a secure box, and there will be someone at the destination to meet and take possession immediately. All these things were set in motion for our bird.

The eagle was given fluids and an antibiotic and placed in a cage where he lay on his side, his maimed feet mute testimony of his fate.

The next morning before appointments began, Marty put the eagle on the operating table and did what he could for it. The toes on one foot were irretrievably lost. The other talons were intact, but the entire foot needed to be sutured back to the ankle. Marty kept shaking his head. "It won't work. This is useless." But he did it anyway, which is the way Marty is. The eagle would be ready to fly on the four o'clock plane out of Central Wisconsin Airport that afternoon.

At about ten o'clock we had a call from the Department of Natural Resources. "Can you take an eagle?" Chet asked. "A guy caught one in a trap out on the Tomahawk River. Says the eagle must have come in for his bait."

"Where is it now?" asked Mark, his heart sinking.

"Right here in the office. He brought it in. It's a mess, I can tell you."

"I'll be right there." said Mark.

And that was the second eagle. This one had been caught by only one foot, and although it was seriously damaged and bleeding profusely, upon examination of it, Marty held out hope. Again Mark called the Raptor Center to tell them that two eagles would arrive on the four o'clock flight, both with trap injuries.

Mark and Dave placed both birds in "eagle boxes" borrowed from the DNR and drove to the Mosinee airport. Then the long wait began. Could either one be saved?

Trappers inspect their traps twice a day by law. Usually this is done in the morning and evening. Since we had heard nothing from the Raptor Center except that the birds had arrived and had been admitted, we closed up at about five-thirty and went home. As was his custom, Dave went back at ten o'clock to check everything one last time and give any necessary treatments.

The Center is never entirely closed to animals. Although the inside door of the foyer is locked, the outside door is left open so

15

that anyone having an injured animal can leave the box in the warm, secure hall until morning. Since darkness, quiet, and safety are all necessary for an injured animal, this is not the worst place in the world for it. Naturally, if there is an emergency, we can be called.

That evening, when Dave returned to the Center, there was a box in the foyer. He carried it to the back room and opened it. Lying on its back, staring up at him, was a third eagle! This was a young one, still with immature plumage, but just as majestic and fierce as the first two...and injured beyond hope. Both legs stuck up, both feet were bloody and hanging loose at the ankle, held only by thin strands of white tendon. Another doomed eagle.

Dave called Mark. Together they did what they could, and the following morning Mark called Pat Redig at the Raptor Center for the third time in two days.

"What's going on over there?" Pat demanded. "You trying to extirpate all the eagles in the state?"

"I don't know," Mark answered. "It's like a horror movie."

This last one was just left in the hall. No name. No nothing.

"Send it over," Pat said wearily. "It doesn't sound good, but we'll have a look."

The third eagle went to Minnesota on the 10:15 plane out of Rhinelander.

Mark turned to Dave. "One is too many, but three is three too many. We have to think of something."

"Try the Audubon Society," Dave suggested, "or the Trappers Association."

"Right," said Mark. "But first the DNR." He picked up the phone and sent out his calls for help.

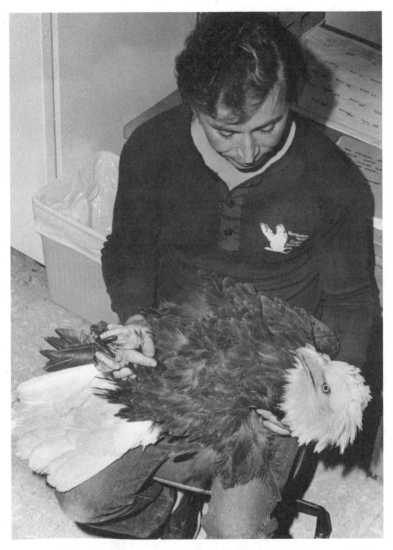

Dave DeBauche holds an injured eagle. Note how he keeps her feet under control; eagle talons are potentially dangerous weapons, and no rehabilitator wants to get "footed."

Ron Eckstein, of the Department of Natural Resources, is the wildlife manager responsible for the bald eagles in the state. He was very much concerned at Mark's call. He called the president of the Wisconsin Trappers' Association, who was also very much concerned. Nobody wanted this to happen. Not only was it illegal to trap birds of prey, but the eagle was an endangered species and every bird counted. Three had now been removed from the population. Assuming that they all came from different territories, two mated pairs had been disrupted, and a young bird had been sacrificed. Even if the birds could be saved to the point of being able to perch, they would never hunt, and would be captive birds for the rest of their lives.

A meeting was called for the following week to discuss the matter and find solutions. Mark and Dave were to attend.

The following day, a fourth maimed and bloody eagle was brought to the Center, not by a trapper, but by a youngster who had found it flapping and screaming, and had called his mother for help. She had wrapped a coat around it, pried open the trap, and carried it in on her lap as she drove the car.

"Do something!" she begged. "Please do something! It's so terribly hurt," and she burst into tears.

Mark patted her on the shoulder, and took the bird. He unwrapped the coat and saw what he had come to expect. Talons damaged beyond repair. He sighed, and reached for the phone. "You're not going to believe this," he told Pat Redig.....

Later, Mark sat with Dave in his office. "This has got to go in the papers," he said. "People have got to know about this."

"You'll have a lot of mad trappers if you make them out the 'bad guys'," Dave said.

"They aren't trying to trap eagles, for Pete's sake. They're trapping for pelts. There's got to be a better way, so that the birds don't see the bait and come in for a free meal."

"Okay. Maybe when they realize what's been happening, they'll think of something. Isn't that what the meeting is about?"

"We need the meeting, but we need something now!" Mark reached for the phone and called the newspaper, the TV stations, and the radio stations. All responded, and the story of the four trapped eagles hit the media with a bang! The fourth eagle was photographed copiously before it was sent to Minnesota. Yet in the two days it took to cover all bases, a fifth trapped eagle was brought to the Center.

"I've caught 'em before, but I didn't know what to do with 'em. I don't want to get fined. I just threw 'em in the woods. This here one, I figured you might fix. He ain't hurt so bad. Just one foot. I seen all that stuff about it on TV, so I brought it in. Big son of a gun, ain't he?"

Marked clamped his jaws tight, and took the eagle, leaving me to cope with the trapper and get the information sheet filled out.

"No way!" the trapper laughed. "I don't put my name on nothing. Just say I brought the bird in." He walked out the door.

His eagle flew to Minnesota the following morning.

That fifth eagle was the last that year....the last brought to the Center. Maybe others were tossed in the woods to die by trappers afraid of a fine, or afraid of censure by their peers, or too busy to be bothered. At the meeting, the consensus was that the Minnesota law whereby bait had to be five feet from the trap itself was a good law and should be adopted by Wisconsin. The fur bearers would walk to the bait and be caught in a trap laid on the periphery of a five-foot circle. A bird, approaching from the air, would be safe.

When it developed that the legislature would be involved, the Center personnel had to withdraw. Lobbying for legislation would jeopardize our nonprofit status. That work had to be left to others. But the law was passed and the raptors were safer.

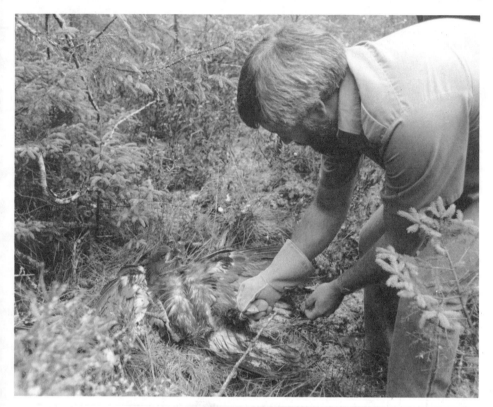

Mark Blackbourn with a young eaglet. Not feeling friendly, the eaglet has flipped onto her back to free her talons for a fight.

The five eagles did not suffer in vain.

In case you are wondering, three had to be euthanized, and two were saved, but would live out their lives in captivity, never to fly free again. You may have seen one of them. Any eagle in captivity is disabled. Healthy birds are in the wild where they were meant to be in the first place.

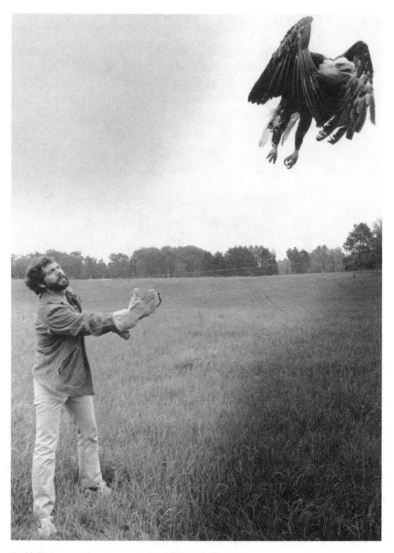

Bill Bauer releases a rehabilitated eagle.

THE LOON EGG

The young people in the power boat were having a lovely time chasing the loons. They had spotted the big birds fishing near a secluded bay and had buzzed them with the boat. The loons had dived and disappeared. The youngsters watched. When the loons surfaced, a shout went up and the driver headed the boat toward them. Again the loons disappeared, to re-emerge moments later farther down the lake. The young people cheered and were soon in pursuit. The harried loons dived again to safety.

By now, others saw what was happening and were angrily standing on their docks yelling and shaking their fists. The youngsters were too intent on their fun to notice. Jim Peters was purple with fury. He knew where the loons' nest was, right in his bay. He had been watching them set their eggs. He spent long hours with binoculars monitoring their safety, relieved every morning that the eggs had not vanished during the night into a predator's stomach. He knew one egg had hatched. The other was still in the nest, now in serious jeopardy if its parents were not there to protect it. Jim started to untie his boat to pursue the pursuers.

The skiers beat him to it. Two young men and two young women had been water skiing when they realized what was happening to the lake's loons. The driver picked up his skier and the others hauled in the rope as the driver headed the boat toward the pursuit boat to head it off. By this time the loons had had enough. They beat their huge wings and slowly raised their heavy bodies out of the water. Airborne at last, they headed toward the other end of the big lake and disappeared.

The ski boat intercepted the youngsters as they turned to follow the loons. There was a near collision, but the ski boat driver was skillful. The youngsters stopped, the boat wallowing in the wakes.

"You kids are beached!" The ski boat driver yelled. "Dock that boat and don't you take it out till past noon tomorrow. Got that?"

The youngsters looked over and started to protest. Then they realized that the skiers were the idols of the lake: Min-Aqua-Bats members of the water ski club that every young skier aspired to. The club performed three nights a week in the Aqua Bowl in Minocqua. Their awe kept them quiet. Four Min-Aqua-Bats in one boat! Each youngster was thinking, "We blew our chance!"

"Dock it NOW!" the ski boat driver repeated. "Or I call the boat patrol."

The youngsters gunned the motor and turned back to shore.

Jim Peters grinned as he watched from his dock. Tension on the lake abated, and Jim walked up to the house for his binoculars to check the egg. It was still there. It was still there two hours later as the sun was going down, alone and unprotected. The loons had not returned. The twilight sky darkened, and Jim was more and more concerned. Finally, he lined a cottage cheese box with a piece of soft worn towel and untied the boat. He rowed around the bay to the opposite shore, and carefully approached the nest. No loons. He gently lifted the egg onto the toweling, and covered it with another piece. Then he rowed back and called Mark at home. The Center was closed.

"Hello," said Mark.

"Guess what I've got?" said Jim.

"Oh, hi, Jim." Mark recognized the voice. "What do you have?"

"I've got a loon egg. What do I do with it?"

"A LOON EGG!" hollered Mark, nearly blasting Jim's ear. "Alive?"

"I think so. Kids chased the adults off the lake and they didn't come back. Left the egg."

Mark was jubilant. "Bring it down. Keep it warm. I'll call Dave. I'll meet you there. Be sure to keep it warm! Not too warm, though! Twenty minutes?"

Jim called his wife. "Sal! Come on. We're taking the egg to the Wildlife Center."

Meanwhile, Mark had been busy. He opened the Center and headed out the back door to gather nesting materials. Dave arrived shortly thereafter. By the time Jim and Sal walked in with their egg, the nest was ready, the incubator light was on and the egg was placed in its new home, safe from all predators. The rescuers went home.

The next morning there were little pecking noises inside the egg. The baby was ready to hatch. This posed a serious problem. Why? A loon is like a chicken. When it hatches and dries into a fluffball, it is ready to go. The loon's parents feed it, but it can swim within hours of hatching. Its eyes are open and alert. The fact that it can see is the problem. When a baby bird of any species once looks around and sees who or what is feeding it, it "imprints" on that image. Since a baby bird usually sees its parents, it imprints on them and is secure in the knowledge of who it is. Mark didn't want the loon chick to imprint on man. When the first hole appeared in the tip of the egg Mark got busy.

"Dave, set up the loon tape on the tape player." Dave did, and soon the rehabilitation room was filled with assorted loon calls. The egg was surrounded with the right sounds. Mark, meanwhile, was on the phone to everyone he knew trying to find a mounted loon to serve as a foster parent. No luck.

He pulled some money out of petty cash and went shopping for a loon statue or carving. He came back in high spirits.

"It's not quite big enough, but it looks right," he said, "and it was the right price. They donated it!" He unwrapped a painted plaster loon and set it on a box next to the nest.

"Not enough," he muttered. "Need something to screen off people."

"How about the posters?" asked Dave.

"Great! Get a couple."

Dave went into the cupboard where the sales items were and brought out two huge loon posters, with which the two men surrounded the egg. The chick could now hatch and take its choice. It could imprint on a smallish plaster parent, or two huge paper ones. It wasn't perfect, but it was something, and certainly better than imprinting on Mark and Dave!

Hours went by. Baby loons take their time. It soon became apparent that it would not be ready for release that day and would have to be held over night.

By the next morning, the nest held a baby loon and some egg shell. The miracle had happened. It was the first hatching of a loon egg in captivity. It was alive and peeping and soon would have to be fed. It was time to find its parents.

Mark called Jim for information.

"Come on up here. The parents are still across the lake, but I found them yesterday and I can find them again today. We'll use my boat."

"We'll bring ours too, and we'll bring Bob Baldwin for pictures." Mark was always alert for public relations, and this was too good to miss.

The entourage set forth about an hour later in two boats. Mark, Dave and the loon in one, and Jim, Sal and Bob Baldwin in the other. It was a long trip across the lake and Mark kept the chick inside his shirt to keep it warm. They searched the far side of the lake.

"There they are! I told you I could find them!" Jim pointed. The others followed his finger to the adult loons and the second chick. "Let's go!"

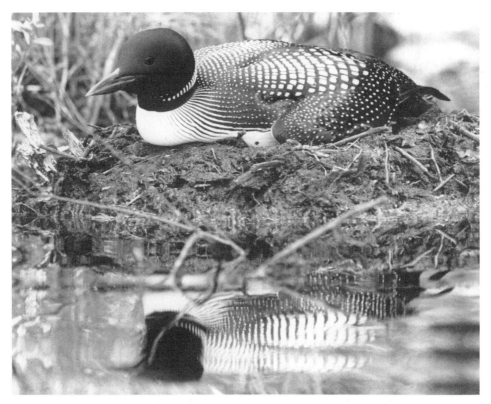

A female loon on her nest. Nests are built close to the water to allow for a quick "getaway," and also to allow the loon, which does not maneuver well on land, easy nest access.

"Sorry, Jim," Mark said. "We don't want to spook them again. Let us take the baby in, and you keep your boat back." Jim was visibly disappointed, but understood. Bob fastened his telephoto lens.

Dave rowed the boat slowly and silently toward the big birds. The loons watched and kept their distance. As the boat approached, the loons seemed to drift away effortlessly.

"This isn't going to work," Mark said. "We'll have to toss the little fellow out." Dave worked the boat as close as possible, and Mark gently removed the chick from his shirt. "Now, when I let him go, you row away fast!" Dave nodded. Mark leaned over the side of the boat and gave a light toss. The little loon landed on the water. Its parents watched as Dave pulled strongly on the oars. Suddenly, the baby loon felt deserted. It turned toward the boat and with a desperate "Peep, peep, peep" it swam to it as fast as its baby legs would go.

"Go back." Mark thought for a moment as the boat returned for the chick. "Ok, this time I'll really toss him." Mark picked up the baby and waited for Dave to get close again. The adults watched this curious pantomime.

This time Mark eased toward the front of the boat and, leaning on the seat and gunwale, he side armed the baby toward its parents. "Go," he said. "Go!" Dave rowed away.

The loon chick was desolate. It was in cold water instead of a warm nest and it headed for security. Back to the boat with its frantic "Peep, peep, peep!" Mark put his head in his hands.

This wasn't going at all well. "Pick him up," he said, and Dave back-paddled to the baby. The adult loons kept their distance and watched.

"Three times and out," said Mark. "This time it's got to work, or we face the fact that he's imprinted!"

"He can't be imprinted," said Dave. "He never got a chance to see us."

"Something's wrong," Mark mourned.

"Heave him out again," Dave said, and rowed back to the loon.

Mark stood up for a major league pitch. As they approached the adults he threw the baby towards its parents. The baby landed with a small squawk. Both adult's heads went up. As Dave back-paddled away, the adults were calling and swimming toward the baby. It peeped and swam to meet them. The parents checked the baby out and decided it was theirs. The people in the two boats watched with lumps in their throats as the baby, after several failures, finally climbed onto the mother's back with its sibling. It was home.

The Wildlife Center had another successful release.

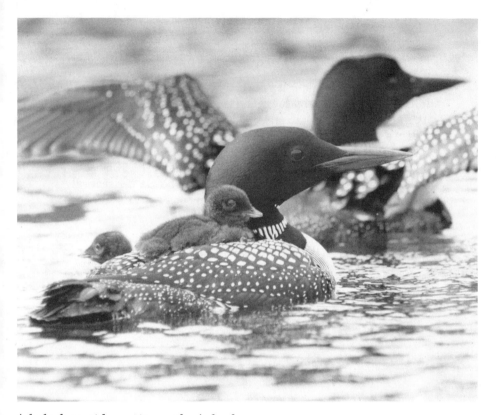

A baby loon rides on its mother's back.

LUMPS IN THE ROAD

"Dangedest thing I ever seen," the old man said, and paused to suck the foam off his mustache. "I come up over a rise and there they was, flopping all over the highway! I never seen nothing like it." He buried his face in his beer mug while the bar regulars waited. They knew a story was coming, but wouldn't give the old man the satisfaction of asking a question. The wait continued as the old man stared into his now empty mug. One of the younger men took pity.

"What happened?" he asked.

"Worth a beer to find out?" the old man asked with a grin.

"Worth a beer," replied the younger man and signaled to the waiting bartender. The bartender grinned as the scenario went on and filled the old man's mug.

"It was a bad night," the old man continued, "snowing like crazy. Bad driving with the flakes coming at you. Couldn't see nothing but a little bit ahead. It was sticking on the shoulders and back in the woods, but not on the road, see? The road was wet and black. The snow was on the sides. Figured they thought it was a river, and come down to rest." He stopped again and stared into his mug. Slowly he lifted it to his lips and took a long pull. "Need to wet my whistle," he explained. "A man gets dry talking."

The younger man was impatient. "What came down to rest? What was it?"

The old man slowly turned to the younger one. "I ain't there, yet." He glared briefly at the questioner and then relaxed. "I come up over this rise, see, and as I come down there's all these lumps on the road in the lights. Another fellow has his car stopped the other way and his headlights blinking. He's stopped. He comes at me waving a light. Flashlight it was. I could barely make him out. I got out of the truck. 'Put your blinker on,' he says. Well now, my old truck, it don't have no blinker, but I turn the plow lights on on the top, and he's happy. 'We got to get them off the road,' the fellow says. I already hit one. I think I killed it,' he says. 'Couldn't stop. They all just came down in front of me. Look at that,' he says. 'There must be a dozen of 'em.'

We walk down the road and count. I'm counting and he's counting, and dinged if we didn't get to 13 of 'em, flopping around and not going any place. Dangedest thing I ever seen." The old man rubbed his hand across his stubbly chin and cheeks, and stared intently at his palm as if reading his future in its rough lines.

Moments passed. One of the regulars shrugged and signaled the bartender. "Fill 'em up," he directed. He turned to the old man. "Emil, this is it. Get to the point, you old mule, or you go dry!"

The old man cradled his brimming mug with both hands and raised it to his lips. After two long swallows, he rubbed his wrist across his mouth and wiped it across his jacket front. "This big sixteen-wheeler come up the road. Reefer, it was. He seen my plowlights and he's down-shiftin' to stop. Just in time, too. Nearly hit the truck. He climbs outen that truck ready for bear cussin' like you woulden want yer ma to hear. I ain't sayin' what he said. It ain't Christian. But he was mad till he seen all them lumps floppin around. Then he ain't mad but he's still cussin to beat all. He climbs back in the truck and CB's the state patrol. He gets out real friendly and ready to talk. Says we done a good thing to stop. Then we all three of us start shooin' them things off the road. But they don't shoo. Seems like they can't go no place on land. They got to have water. They're flappin' their wings and scooting along on their bellies and getting nowheres. Dangedest thing I ever seen. Pretty soon Smoky comes along with his siren blowing to scare the insides outen them things, but they just siren back at him. You never heard such a ruckus in your born days. Like a crazy house, it was." The old man paused, remembering, shaking his head in wonder.

"Don't stop!" the young man said menacingly. "Don't you dare stop! He's eggin' for another beer! Where does it go?"

Angered, the old man bristled. "I ain't eggin' for a beer. I'm figuring how to tell the rest. I got a right to figure how to tell it, ain't I?"

"OK, OK. Figure! But hurry up about it! We ain't got all night, Emil. Let's get on with it."

Thus prodded by one of the regulars, Emil gave up on his hope for additional refreshment, and headed for a quick conclusion.

"Smoky seen what was going on and he headed back to his radio and called the wardens. That's the DNR guys. They come next with nets and boxes and caught 'em and took 'em away. That's all." He started to fasten his heavy red plaid jacket with complete unconcern.

"What were they?" The young man yelled. "Tell us what they were!"

The old man turned to leave. "Swallow yer tongue, young feller. Them was loons."

"Loons?"

"Loons." As the old man spoke, there was silence as the men contemplated the vision of thirteen loons on US 51.

"Son of a gun," breathed one of the regulars. "That's a new one." He frowned. "Didn't think they migrated in flocks."

"Don't," answered the old man. "Them was young ones. First time, and they botched it. Old ones go first. Foller the river or go from lake to lake. These ones follered the road. Once they come down, they was done for."

"Why? Why done for?" asked the young man. The old man had regained his complete attention.

"Can't take off from land. They gotta have water they can run across. Maybe quarter mile before they git up."

"What happened? Where'd they take them?" The young man asked.

The old man was in his glory. "To the hospital, of course. Where'd you think? I follered the wardens," he said slowly and deliberately. "They took them loons to the hospital. I was there. I seen it. I seen the doctors. I seen 'em takin' all them loons in, all thirteen boxes, even the dead one, they took. I heered 'em talking X-rays and shots. I seen it all myself, with these here eyes. How about that, young feller?" He waited a moment. "Worth a beer?" The young man bought.

That was the night the Department of Natural Resources wardens brought thirteen stranded loons to the Wildlife Center. Naturally, we were closed and when the DNR called Mark Blackbourn, the director, Mark called Dave Debauche, the rehabilitator, and the two of them got ready to receive some new patients. By the time they had opened the building and prepared the back room for business, the loons were arriving. Box by box, they were brought in, while everyone marveled that they were still alive after their crash landings.

Each bird was examined carefully for injuries, particularly wings and "knee bones" and legs. Any that were questionable were set aside for X-rays. All were given shots for shock and an antibiotic to combat any infection as all the birds had scraped their feet in landing and had bleeding abrasions which had to be cleaned and treated. Mark and Dave soon had an assembly line set up, including the wardens. The most deadly weapon on a loon is its beak. It is long and sharp and incredibly quick. It has to be to catch a fish dinner underwater. Anyone trying to treat a loon has to control its beak with one hand, tuck the wings into its body and under the other arm to hold them there. That does not leave much extra to use for medicating or giving shots. It's definitely a two-man job. Since the wardens were experienced, they did the holding and Mark and Dave did the treating.

The "completed" loons were returned to the dark security of their boxes to recover from shock. Only one proved to be in serious trouble. The one with the broken beak. He must have landed face down. He, too, was placed in a dark box for the night. Before work could begin on his beak, he had to be stabilized. Injured and captured birds experience an accelerated heart rate and must be calmed down before they can be anesthetized and operated on.

When the birds were safely back in their boxes, the men cleaned up and headed out the front door. They found an old man waiting patiently in one of the chairs in the visitors area.

"I wasn't asleep," he assured them. "Just restin' like, waitin' to see how them birds come out. Dangedest thing I ever seen. There they was floppin' around on the road..." Mark explained about the treatment. The old man nodded knowingly, understanding only half through a haze of sleep, but he was blissful to be a part of this adventure. He could imagine how it would be. How he would tell the story.

"Dangedest thing I ever seen," he muttered as he went out the door to his truck.

Eleven of the loons were released the next morning to continue their migration. We hope they made it. They would remain in the south until they grew their adult plumage two years later. Only then would they return to claim a territory and mate.

The twelfth loon, with the broken beak, was literally glued back together. The break was outside the "live" area where tiny blood vessels nourish its growth — just as your fingernail may break above the "quick." Epoxy glue put him back together again, but although he seemed fine, and was happily eating minnows in the pond, he apparently had other injuries. Two mornings later when we came in, he had died. No, we still don't know why.

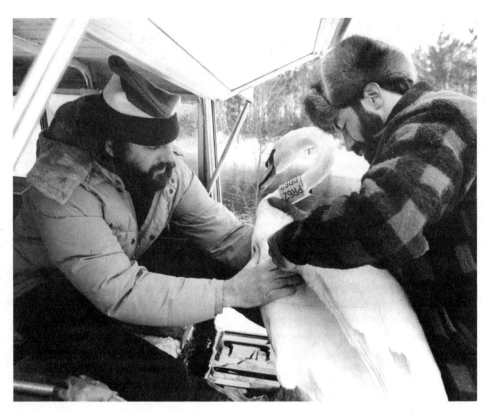

Mute swan "PR-62" arrives at the Center in the care of Bill Bauer and a DNR ranger.

PR-62

The swans lay sleeping with their majestic necks curled to the side and their heads warm under their wings. Only the cob was awake and standing sentinel duty. The sleeping swans looked like floating blobs of whipped cream, some of which had washed up on shore. To the female coyote, they looked delicious and she was hungry. Belly down, she crept along behind the brush growing above the high water mark, her dun coat blending in with the dun-colored growth. The wind was off Lake Superior and carried her scent away. The waves masked any noise she might have made. She had only to make the short run across the bare sand. It looked like an easy meal, and her heart was beating fast.

The cob stretched his neck and shook his feathers straight. He ran one between his beak to smooth it, and settled back down on the sand. A glance around the area showed nothing amiss. He tested the air. Nothing.

Suddenly there was a small brown explosion on the bank, and faster than light the female coyote dove for one of the sleeping swans. The swan awoke and squawked just as the cob started down the shore, his wings flapping hugely as he sprang to the defense of one of his flock. The female coyote suddenly felt very small, but was determined to fight for her dinner.

She turned to face the oncoming cob, and to her intense dismay, the bird she thought she had caught flew away. Then all the white mounds came alive and flew out to the safety of the waters of Lake Superior! About to withdraw from the fray, the disappointed coyote turned only to find herself strongly pummeled by the heavy wing beats of the cob. Desperate, she sprang at him, teeth slashing. She bowled him over backwards, and then jumped on one outstretched wing while he was out of action, and made her escape. Dinner that night was mouse, not swan.

The cob struggled upright, but something was terribly wrong

with one wing. For safety he made for the water, but he couldn't fly. He walked into the shallows and finally was floating. The wing throbbed and did not fold properly along his side and back. He preened his feathers, but that was no help. He pecked at the wing but that only increased the pain. Finally, he accepted what was his lot, and endured, as all animals do.

The Wisconsin Department of Natural Resources was interested in reintroducing the trumpeter swan into the state. Before this could be done, it was necessary to be sure that they would be able to survive in the current environment. Among other preparations, the lead levels in the blood of existing mute swan populations would have to be tested and evaluated, since lead poisoning had been a problem among other waterfowl in the state. The research project started with the Ashland mute swan flock. Among the researchers was Bill Bauer, then executive director, of the Wildlife Center.

The mute swan is far from mute, making a variety of different sounds, depending upon the circumstances. It is not a native bird, but was introduced from Europe in the early 1800's as a captive bird with clipped wings, which enhanced the beauty of many small ponds on large estates. As all wild things will if given a chance, some escaped, found each other, and multiplied. The flocks started in the east and south, but gradually worked their way across the country. Why the Ashland flock chose the harsh environment of northern Wisconsin, no one knows. But they have been there for years. When the lake freezes, the flock migrates to the open Trout River near Manitowish Waters, not more than a hundred miles south. There, they seem to prefer the water near a small bridge, and are easily viewed by resident swan lovers.

The research party started at Ashland. One by one the frightened swans were netted, and collars were placed around their necks for identification. The wide yellow collar around the neck of the cob read PR-62. Small blood samples were taken, and the swans were released. They would be tested again at the end of the summer.

However, when the researchers re-tested the swans at the Trout River location in the fall, PR-62 was nowhere to be found. For some reason, he had not migrated with the flock. Dead?

Then the Center received a phone call from Ashland.

"There's a swan up here with ice around his neck" the caller said. "He can't fly."

"We'll be right up!" said Bill. He called to Dave and the two of them drove to Ashland to rescue the swan. The caller provided a boat and it was no problem to catch the bird since it was exhausted and frightened at the heavy weight around its neck. Of course, it was PR-62! Because he remained in the water for safety, ice had formed and had gradually built up into a huge ice collar that was unmanageable. Bill and Dave thanked the caller and took PR-62 back to the Center to melt.

"Dave, look at this." Bill called. "He is all clear of the ice, but he looks awkward. Something — look here, his wing."

Dave carefully extended the huge right wing. "You're right. It's not straight. Let's get an X-ray." He picked up PR-62 and carried him next door to the hospital. Sure enough, the X-ray revealed an old break, now healed, but with a large calcium deposit so close to the 'elbow' that the wing could not be fully extended.

"Shot?" asked Bill.

"Maybe, but it doesn't look like it. Fight, maybe. Swans fight for dominance and for territory. Could have been in a fight." Dave surmised. He set the X-ray down. "If he doesn't fly, he'll have trouble surviving the winter. He couldn't escape from a predator, and he'll end up with another ice build up. We better keep him here. I'll call the DNR."

PR-62 spent that winter in our courtyard. This worked out well for the trumpeter swan research team as well, since PR-62, living and feeding outside of his natural environment, could be used as a control in monitoring the lead levels in the flock's blood.

PR-62 started out with a blood level of .88 parts per million, which is relatively high. Where were the swans getting the lead? It was assumed that they were ingesting it in pellet form! They were eating the water plants near the bridge during the winter. This is a favorite spot for fishermen in the summer. Lead sinkers lost in the summer were being swallowed by the swans in the winter. Research on one dead swan found not only death by lead poisoning, but a telltale sinker in his digestive tract. Either the bridge area would have to be closed to fishing with lead sinkers, or the swans would have to learn to winter in a safer place.

In the spring, when the swan flock returned to Lake Superior, the DNR picked up PR-62 to return him to his friends and relatives. Since he was the dominant cob in the flock, he was needed to perform his breeding duties. After a life of ease and luxury at Hotel Wildlife Center, he was in excellent shape. He may not have been able to fly, but he was not otherwise handicapped.

The following fall, when the swans returned to the Trout River, again, no PR-62. And again we had a call about a swan in trouble on Lake Superior. This time, picking him up was a tough job. Ice had already formed, and a boat had to be pushed out on the ice to the open water where PR-62 was floating forlornly. Finally, after a dunking in a wet suit, Dave was able to net his swan, and PR-62 was again a Wildlife Center resident.

He was dried out and warmed up in the flight room. Blood samples were taken and his lead level had gone down to .24 PPM, a significant drop, almost confirming the sinkers as the source of lead poisoning in the swans. PR-62 did not have any. His lead level dropped.

"I don't remember the lump on his wing being that big, do you?" Bill said as he and Dave watched PR-62 through the one-way glass.

"No," said Dave and went into the room. After a brief scuffle, he had the swan tucked under his arm, right wing out for examination. "Much bigger," Dave agreed. "Time for another X-ray."

He carried the huge bird down the hall and a short time later returned him to the flight room. He and Bill went back to develop the film. The resulting picture was both disheartening and infuriating.

"Look at that!" Dave said angrily. "A .22 pellet! Some stinker shot a sitting swan!"

"No way he could have been flying!" agreed Bill. "No one could say he made a mistake! This is a deliberate aim and fire! Target shooting at a helpless live bird! Who would be that rotten?"

"Had to have been shot broadside to hit that spot that way. I'd like to get my hands on that great sportsman just for five minutes!"

"He's really helpless, now." Bill said as he and Dave went back to the flight room window. "What a shame."

Once again, PR-62 spent the winter in the courtyard. Since he defended the courtyard as his territory, there was hardly a volunteer who escaped without a warning pinch on the leg from the big yellow bill sometime during that winter. Injured or not, PR-62 was still very much the 'head man'.

In the spring, the DNR came to take him back to Ashland.

"What do you think? Will he make it?" Chet asked.

"Hard to say," replied Dave. "If he stays close to the water, he should have no problem. Nothing wrong with his feet. But, if he gets too far away from the water, anything could get him. He needs to be where he can swim out of danger."

"How about it? Do we take him back to the lake, or put him down?"

"I'd hate to put him down. Let him have a good summer and take his chances," said Dave. "We'll see about next winter."

WILDLIFE HOSPITAL

PR-62 went back to Ashland with his flock for the summer on Lake Superior.

In the fall, when the swans returned to the river, as usual, there was no PR-62. Our caller, who watched the swans, did not call. There was no word of PR-62.

"It's a nice day," said Bill. "Feel like a ride?"

Dave grinned. "To Ashland?"

Bill smiled back. "I sort of had that in mind."

"You're on," said Dave and picked the truck keys off the rack.

They stopped where they had found the big cob previously. No swan. They walked the shore all along the area where the swans spent the summer raising their little cygnets, eating the water plants and small grubs of aquatic animals, where they sunned themselves with wings outstretched, where they swam in the blue water, where they preened their white feathers, where they slept like blobs of whipped cream on the shore with one sentinel awake and watchful. The swans had left now. The waters had turned green, and were beginning to freeze on the edges. Cold winds cut through the two walking men. They walked more and more slowly, and then stopped.

"We'd better head back," said Bill.

"Guess so," agreed Dave.

PR-62 was gone.

THE UNEXPECTED HAPPENS

We don't know what happened to him, but when he was brought in, the porcupine was a mess! He had a jagged tear down the center of his underside which ran from the top of his chest all down his stomach. Blood was everywhere in the box he came in.

One does not treat a porcupine carelessly. Dave put on heavy gloves and gingerly picked him up. The extent of the injury made this an immediate emergency. Dave took him next door to Marty. Happily, it was near lunch time and there were no clients at the animal hospital. The operating room was set up and the big lights turned on. The bristling porky was given a tranquilizer first to calm him down and then he was anesthetized.

"Wow, look at that!" Marty said as he was able to get a better look at the now still little animal. "Something ripped him right down the middle."

"What?" asked Dave. "What could do that? A dog?"

"No dog. A bobcat, maybe. Or maybe he got hung up on a barbed wire fence. It's deeper than that, though." Marty's hands were busy with the sutures. "Guess we'll never know."

"Quills all over." Dave picked one up. "They've got barbs on the ends. Like a fishhook." Dave examined it closely.

"Ever get one in you?" asked Marty.

"No, but I've taken them out of my dog. Had to use pliers."

"The barbs keep working into the animal. Every time he moves, the quills go deeper. Terrific design for defense. Even after the attack, the weapons keep working." Marty kept sewing the wound. The little knots with their neatly cut ends made a parade down the center of the porky's abdomen. "There, that should do him." Marty took off his gloves. "Keep him on Amoxy, and he should be OK. I'll look in later."

Dave put the welder's gloves back on and picked up his patient holding him tummy-side-up as he carried him back down the hall to the back room cages. The porky remained hospitalized for the ten days it took before the stitches could be removed.

When the stitches were out, we put him in an outside cage which had a tree in it and gave him a chance to recover his climbing skills. The porcupine knew better than to subject his tender tummy to the rough bark of a tree. He remained on the ground. Dave tempted him by putting his food a short way up. The porky went hungry before he would climb. It began to look as if he could not go back into the wild after all. Gloom descended. All the work and all the TLC was to go down the drain. Now, mind you, we do not make pets of the patients. But somehow, when you have an animal here for any length of time, you become attached. The idea of euthanizing the porcupine was a horror!

Fate stepped in. A man from the Milwaukee Museum called and asked whether we had an unreleasable porcupine. Theirs had died and they needed a replacement for their summer education program.

"He'd be well cared for," the man promised. "He'd be at the museum in the summers and will winter at the Milwaukee Zoo."

"Fine," said Bill happily. "We just happen to have what you are looking for. We'll arrange permission to transfer him."

The porcupine had received his reprieve. Now at this time, the non-climbing porky was ensconced outside in our courtyard where he had lots of room for walking around on the grass and weeds, nibbling this and that. He was on display through the one-way window. Bill's office was one of the walls of the courtyard, and we are quite sure that the porky heard the entire conversation. The phone call came on a Monday. The museum man would pick up the porky the following Sunday.

THE UNEXPECTED HAPPENS

On Thursday when we came to work, the porky was GONE! No sign of him anywhere. Dave, Bill, and the volunteer began searching the woods. Since we have a lot of property, it took a while before the escapee was found back by the pine marten cages. He had climbed the big pine tree in the courtyard, gone over the roof and climbed down the other side. Then he took off through the woods. No museum life for him! He was going back into the wild!

We marked his chart "Released."

So far as we know, he still lives in our woods.

SNOWY OWL

The huge snowy owl ranged over the arctic tundra like a giant snowflake, and just as silently. She needed food and her prey had disappeared. The lemmings upon which she preyed had undertaken a mass migration to the west. Urged on by some mindless instinct, they scurried across the landscape, oblivious to obstacles and unable to stop or turn. Whatever their final destiny, they had left the area. The owl had found a mouse or two in the last few days and was desperate for food. She turned south.

Out of the arctic she flew, finding just enough small rodents to keep her going. She spent time in Canada, but as she hunted, she kept drifting to the south. Food was not plentiful, and some days she felt herself weakening. A lucky kill would sustain her for a while, but she was losing weight and strength, and hunting became more difficult. She was slow and clumsy now, and less successful. She flew around the end of Lake Superior into Wisconsin. Fresh snows along the lake made hunting even more difficult. She pumped her tired wings still southward. Exhaustion overcame her. Silently she glided to the forest floor, landing in the snow near a small pine tree. It was a week before Christmas.

"Today's the day!" Greg Watkins called up the stairs. "I'm going out to find a Christmas tree! Do I have any helpers?" He waited.

"Me!"

"Me!"

"Me!"

The response was all Greg could have wished as his three children came tumbling down the stairs in their pajamas.

"Hey, there! Just a minute! I'm not taking three pairs of pajamas. Everybody back upstairs and get dressed. Then breakfast first.

Have to have fuel to stoke your inside furnaces. Right?" He patted the bottom of the last pair of pajamas up the stairs. It was going to be a great day. He turned and hugged Chrissie, his wife.

"You, too?"

"Wouldn't miss it for the world!"

When the family was all fed and dressed in sufficient snow pants, scarves, mittens and boots to brave the northern Wisconsin winter, Greg herded them all into the car and they were off to cut their own Christmas tree. Greg had a permit to cut in a forty acre tract some ten miles north of town. He had surveyed the situation a few days ago and had several possibilities already selected. He didn't want to keep the children out too long in the cold winter morning.

"Here we are!" he said happily. "Everybody out!"

The children exploded from the car into the woods, suddenly floundering in the deep snow. They fell down and giggled, stood up and fell down again on purpose until they were covered with white frosting and only their pink cheeks showed.

"They are going to be soaked," Chrissie murmured in a low voice. "We'd better make a quick pick."

"There's a path over here. C'mon kids, this way. Follow the leader." He began an erratic trek down the path with jumps, hops, short runs and elephant walks, with the children behind keeping up the best they could. Chrissie helped Teeny, the littlest, whose proper name was Christine, after her mother. Teeny had a hard time with the leader game, but she was grinning broadly as her mother bounced her along behind the others.

It wasn't long before they came to a small clearing and Greg's first possibility.

"How about this one?" he asked, panting a bit.

The children examined it carefully. The older ones knew there were more to come. They weren't going to make a too-quick decision and spoil the rest of the fun.

"No! Not this one," said Mark.

"No. Not big enough," said Trish. "What's next?"

Chrissie played her part. "This is fine. Let's cut it and go home."

"NO!" shouted all the children. "Find another, Daddy."

"This way," said Greg, and headed down a path that forked to the left. There were many small pines in the tract. Because they needed to be thinned out, the owner had set up a Christmas tree cut. As they walked along, they passed many suitable trees, but that was not part of the game. Greg's next tree was a bit larger than the first, stood by itself so that it had developed branches on all sides. It definitely had possibilities.

"There! How about this one?" he asked triumphantly.

"It will never fit in the living room!" exclaimed Chrissie, not playing a part this time. "It's huge!"

Greg looked abashed. "I wasn't thinking about that, I guess." He winked at Chrissie. "It's probably about ten, twelve feet. Guess it wouldn't fit after all. My mistake. We'll have to look at my last pick."

Actually, Greg had known that that tree was not for cutting. Other trees had been taken out around it to allow it to develop properly. This was exactly why the Christmas tree cut had been arranged. He moved on down the path. "Side-step!" he directed.

The children side-stepped after him, Teeny, with Chrissie's help. She was getting tired, and was beginning to feel cranky. Her lower lip began to stick out, and her mouth turned down at the corners.

"Here we are!" said Greg. "The best of the best! They don't grow any better than this one! Just look at those branches! Think of our angel on the top!"

The children looked. It was undeniably THE TREE. They were excited and awed. Then they shouted.

"This is the one! I pick this one! I pick this one!" Again they began to play in the snow. Teeny fell and got snow down her neck. For her that was the last straw.

"I don't want that old tree!" she screamed. "I want this one!" she ran to scraggly little pine and threw herself down next to it. "This one! This one! This one!" She kicked her heels and made a dreadful scene. Suddenly, she screamed a genuine scream. "There's something here. There's something here!" She struggled to get up out of the snow in panic. "Daddy! Daddy!"

Greg ran over and scooped her up. "There, now, it's all right. There's nothing there. It's all right, Baby Doll. There, there."

"There is, too, something there!" shouted Mark. "It's a bird. A big bird!" He left the area in a big enough hurry to get out of harm's way, but not so fast as to be construed a bolt.

Greg gave Teeny to her mother and went to investigate. The children were right. It was a huge snowy owl. It had been there a while from the looks of things. No visible damage. Maybe he could have it stuffed for the mantle. Chrissie loved owls. This would make a good "after-Christmas" present. He carried the limp bird to show the others.

"Probably starved to death. There's not a mark on it. It couldn't have been attacked by anything. Look at that wing span!" He extended one of the wings.

"It's beautiful!" breathed Chrissie.

"If you have been a particularly good wife this year, Santa might have it stuffed for you." Greg grinned.

49

"Oh, I have, Santa. I'd love it." Chrissie was ecstatic.

"What about the tree?" wailed Trish. "We need to get our tree!"

"My tree! My tree!" Teeny yelled.

"Teeny, look at this. Come here and look. It's all right. I put the bird down by the ax and the rope. Come here."

Teeny walked to Greg.

"See the top of this little tree? It's a porcupine tree. When it was little, a hungry porcupine came along and ate the top off. The tree had to make some changes in how it was going to grow. Two of the upper side branches began to grow up, instead of out, to be the new top. That's the way a little pine tree makes up for having its top eaten. With two tops, a porcupine tree isn't right for our angel. See?"

Teeny was adamant. "I want the owl tree. I found it. It's my tree."

"Yes, we should have the owl tree," said Trish, "to remind us of our adventure."

"Oh, come on!" scoffed Mark. "Who wants an old porcupine tree!"

"It's not a porcupine tree! It's an owl tree! And it's mine!" screamed Teeny.

"Oh, have your owl tree," agreed Mark grudgingly. "Who cares. We can put two ornaments on the top. We'll have twice as many as anybody." He showed off his arithmetic.

Greg looked at Chrissie. She nodded. "Ok, the Porcupine-owl tree it is. Everybody stand back while I chop." He picked up his ax and chopped at the tree.

The owl lay quiet. Not a muscle moved.

The family hike back to the car was not as exuberant as the hike in. Greg was burdened with the tree and the owl. Chrissie was carrying Teeny, and Mark and Trish were tired. When they got to the car, the tree and the owl went into the trunk and the lid was fastened down with rope.

When the family got home the tree went into the house to be set up and trimmed. The owl stayed in the trunk of the car to wait through the weekend until Greg could get to the taxidermist.

Again, the owl lay quiet, not moving.

On Monday, on his way to work, Greg stopped at the taxidermist and took the owl inside.

"I'd like to have this stuffed for my wife. We found it in the woods when we went for a Christmas tree."

The taxidermist was examining the bird as Greg talked. He looked up at Greg intently.

"Mister, there's two reasons I can't stuff this bird for you. One is, you don't have a permit, and the other is this bird's alive."

Greg's mouth dropped. "Alive?" he gasped. "All this time alive?"

"Sure's your breathing, so is he. Here, feel." He placed Greg's hand on the owl's breast. "Feel it?"

"I think so." Greg said softly. "Now what do I do?"

"If I were you, I'd take him to the Wildlife Center. Maybe they could bring him back. It's out on Highway 70 West in Minocqua."

"I go that way to work. I'll stop in." Greg reached for the owl. The taxidermist held on for a moment while looking hard at Greg.

"Yes, I guess you'll get there. I'd be breaking the law letting you take a live owl out of here if you weren't taking it to the hospital. I don't want any trouble."

"You won't have any. I promise. I'll take him right over."

Greg arrived at the Wildlife Center shortly after it opened at eight. He explained about the owl and delivered it into the capable hands of Dave DeBauche.

Dave took the owl into the rehab area and laid it gently on the treatment table. Fluids first, he thought as he carefully felt the owls keel bone. A starving owl's keel bone looks like the breast bone of your Thanksgiving turkey on the day you consign it to the soup kettle. No meat on it at all. The snowy owl was all skin and feathers. She weighed about a third of her normal weight. With the help of Tony, who was managing the Center, Dave gave the owl two sources of fluids: subcutaneously via injection, and via tube directly down her throat. The fluids were chosen to give the maximum nutrition, the necessary stimulants, plus the electrolytes the owl needed to keep her alive. After he had treated her, he placed her in a cage on her side on a soft towel. Under the towel, he put a special heating pad turned on low.

All through the day, Dave alternated the fluids and the warming. Marty kept checking the owl's vital signs between his vet patients at the clinic next door. He reported that the owl's kidneys had shut down, and the prognosis was poor. She had been too long without food. Dave continued to work with her. Tony brought him a cheeseburger and a malt, and he stayed with the owl through the day.

"C'mon, baby, C'mon," he coaxed. "Respond a little. Let's see a twitch."

The owl lay quiet. At eleven-thirty at night, her heart fluttered, her wing muscles contracted, her eyes opened wide, and then shut again as the fluttering heart stopped. Dave held her in his hands, and blinked his own eyes which had become suddenly blurry.

"Damn," he said. "Damn."

He tied a toe tag on her and put her in the freezer. Then he turned to her chart, picked up a pen and checked the square after "deceased."

He washed his hands and wiped them on a paper towel, then quickly, with the towel, he wiped his face.

"Damn," he said, and went out the door locking it as the chimes from a nearby church marked midnight.

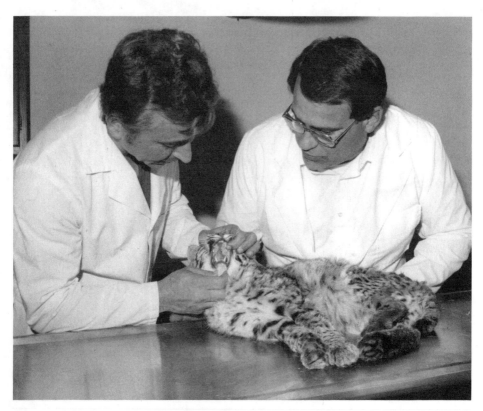

Dave and Warren examine the bobcat's teeth to check her age and determine that she's only a youngster.

THE BOBCAT'S STORY

The bobcat flew through the air upon impact. With a "thump" she landed in the roadside ditch and lay still. The car that hit her slowed momentarily and then accelerated into the distance. The mouse the bobcat had been chasing vanished into the tall grasses, grateful that fate had saved him one more time.

When the bobcat regained her senses, she was still in shock and thought she was still in pursuit of her prey. Her first reaction was to continue the chase, but nothing came together right for her. Her back legs would not work at all. Suddenly the pain washed over her, and she was again unconscious. For the rest of the night, she drifted in and out of consciousness. In the morning, instinct took over, and she had a strong need to find cover.

Dragging her body by her front legs, she pulled herself out of the ditch. After this exertion, she rested. Again, using only her front legs, she slowly and painfully crept to some bushes surrounding the outbuildings of a farmyard. It was a long and painful trip, made with frequent pauses, but her fear of exposure overrode her pain, and she finally achieved her goal: cover for the day surrounded by brush. She slept.

When evening came, she was frantic for water. She raised her muzzle to the breeze. Her sensitive nose told her water was near, but when she tried to move, her body was stiff and sore, and utterly immobile from the hips back. Again, she had to drag herself in the direction of the small brook which ran through the farm field. Her desperate need kept her moving until she could bury her muzzle in the cool water. She drank her fill, lying at full length on the brook's bank.

Exposed as she was after her drink, she slept again. Other animals came to drink, among them an unwary meadow vole which happened along just as the bobcat awoke. "Whack!" went a lightening-swift paw, and the vole was dinner, the first food the bobcat had had since her accident. The vole only stimulated her appetite, but no other prey came within reach, and she decided she had to look elsewhere.

She pulled her body back the way she had come toward the cover of the bushes. In the farmyard itself, there were numerous mouse holes in the ground and near roots of grass clumps. The bobcat could hardly believe her good luck! She chose a place between two holes and waited. Near her, but out of reach, she watched as a kangaroo mouse nosed around and gathered seeds. Once loaded, the mouse jumped away and into one of the holes. Then, small noises arose from one of the holes near her. The bobcat lay still with every muscle poised for attack. The scrabbly noise came closer and the bobcat tried to set her back legs for a spring. They would not work. She winced with the pain of the attempt and the field mouse left his hole and went out of reach. The bobcat waited. After gathering his supply of seeds, the field mouse started to return to his hole, but his nose told him something was amiss, and he had better choose a different hole for storing his collection. He ran off to the right of the strange new smell, but he underestimated the reach of the swift paw which scooped him up to a waiting mouth. The bobcat shook the mouse once and gulped.

During the long night, she was successful only one more time. It was not enough for her fifteen pounds, but it was something. As the light broke, she again sought cover for the daylight hours behind the outbuilding and in the bushes.

And so she lived, halfstarving, but still surviving, until one morning when she was late in seeking cover.

"Roger! Come here quick! Look out there, under the bird feeder! Isn't that a bobcat?" Joyce Boggs called to her husband.

Roger came running.

"You're right! That's just what it is! Son of a gun! I haven't seen one of those in years!"

"What do you suppose it's doing right out there in the yard? They never come around people!"

Roger shrugged. "Beats me," he said. "Wait! Look!"

Both looked out at the bobcat slowly dragging itself across the yard.

"Oh, the poor thing! It's hurt!" Joyce exclaimed. "What can we do?"

"We can't do anything! Hurt, or not, I'm not messing with a bobcat. I'll call the DNR and let them handle it!" He turned toward the phone.

"I'll watch it. Oh, it's going away." Joyce ran for the door and stood on the porch to see where the bobcat went. She watched it drag its body around the machine shed and out of sight. Slowly, she went down the porch steps and followed until she could again see the bobcat. She watched as it crawled under the bushes and lay quiet.

"He said they'd be right over. I had to call Bill at home. Where is he?" Roger had come out on the porch.

"Behind the shed. Let's leave him. He's not going anywhere. Come in and get your breakfast." Joyce started for the house. Roger waited for her.

"Wonder what happened to the poor guy," he said as they went through the door into the big farm kitchen.

"Oh, the sausages!" cried Joyce, grabbing the frying pan from the burner. "They're ruined!"

"Never mind! It isn't every day we get a bobcat in the back yard," Roger consoled her. "We'll skip sausage today." He settled comfortably in his chair at the table. It was not a typical dining room chair. It was upholstered and soft and had arms to lean on. It was good for eating, and good for just sitting, sipping coffee and

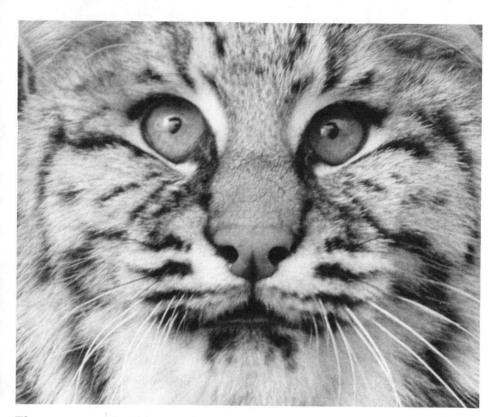

The now-tranquilized bobcat. Nice kitty!

talking. He wouldn't use anything else. Today, he was not disposed to start the farm work until the bobcat was taken care of.

"Wonder what they'll do with him," he mused. "Hope they don't shoot him. He's pretty bad though. Seemed like he couldn't use those back legs at all."

"Don't even say that! I wish we hadn't called them, if they are going to shoot him." Joyce was plainly upset.

"We just have to wait and see. You wouldn't want him just to suffer and die now, would you?"

"No. I guess not," Joyce admitted.

"We'll just have to wait and see. They'll do the right thing. Now don't you fret." Roger patted Joyce's hand across the table. She gave him a halfsmile, and they sat quietly drinking their coffee.

After a while a car drove into the driveway. Doors slammed and Joyce and Roger stepped out on the porch to meet Bill Meier from the Merrill DNR ranger station. Bill was tall and blond with an open, friendly face. Joyce felt reassured immediately. This nice young man wouldn't shoot anything!

"Hi! Understand you have a bobcat," Bill Meier said. "What happened?"

"We don't know what happened. We just saw him out the window this morning early," Roger said. "Joyce saw him first. She followed him. She can show you where he is."

"This is my partner and right hand man, Bruce Klaes. Joyce and Roger Boggs." Bill introduced the second man climbing out of the truck. After greeting, the rangers got their equipment from the truck and turned to Joyce. "Lead the way. We're ready," Bill said, and followed Joyce.

The men walked around behind the shed. The bobcat was alert, but unable to flee. She raised up on her front legs and snarled. She used her most frightening growls and spittings, but still the humans came closer. She was terrified, helpless and surrounded.

One of the men produced a catch-pole. This consisted of a noose on the end of a long pole. The noose could be made larger and smaller by manipulating the handle. The man brought it close to her face. She lashed out, but he whipped the noose out of reach. Slowly, he brought it back. As he moved, he spoke reassuringly.

"It's all right, fella, it's all right. Just hold still. We'll get some help for you. Hold still now. Softly, softly....Whoops!" He took the pole out of reach again.

The bobcat watched him suspiciously, not understanding the words, but understanding that the tone was not threatening.

Once again, the man brought the noose closer, talking quietly. Another man moved on the right, momentarily distracting the bobcat's attention. In a flash, the noose was around her neck and tightened enough to hold her. The bobcat fought mightily as best she could in her disabled condition, but the noose held her head close to the ground. She felt her hindquarters being lifted onto something and held there.

The rangers had placed a heavy cardboard under her and tied her hindquarters with straps to immobilize them for the journey to the hospital. Then, noose, stretcher, cat and all were transported through the yard to the truck and placed in a carrier. Once she was safely inside, the noose was released and the door shut. She flared out the wire mesh window and snarled, starting a loud protest that would last twenty-five miles to the Wildlife Hospital.

Alerted by Bill Meier, Dave and Bill were ready to receive the bobcat. Heavy gloves were on the back counter, and the tranquilizer solution was in the syringe. Dave had even called Bob Baldwin, and he was ready with his camera. The arrival of the bobcat was an EVENT!

When the truck arrived, everyone ran outside. Bill and Dave

unloaded the spitting cat in its carrier, and Bob took a picture of the outraged bobcat through the wire mesh. Since the cat had been put in the carrier head first, the rump was nearest the door which was very handy for injecting the tranquilizer. Then came the wait. The men stood around the truck while Bill told about the capture. From time to time, they would inspect the bobcat. It was not long before she settled down and became quiet. Bob took another picture of a bobcat that looked like somebody's loved pet. The change was dramatic.

The cat was gently removed from the carrier and taken to the treatment room to be examined. It was obvious that her back legs were fractured. She was carried into the Foster-Smith Hospital and X-rayed. Eyes wide open, but calm and quiet, she lay on the X-ray table while Dave positioned her. In a few minutes the entire series of radiographs was taken and she was returned to the Wildlife Center and put in a cage in the cage room.

When the radiographs were developed, the entire Center team and the vets at the animal hospital looked them over, holding one after the other up to the light, shaking their heads and exclaiming softly about what a mess she was. Both hind legs had several fractures and her left hip had been shattered. No doubt the impact had resulted in some internal injuries as well. Her future looked dim....and brief.

"What do you think?" Dave asked the vets. "Put her down?"

"With any other animal I would, but she is a cat. They heal," Marty said. He looked at the others. "How about it? Shall we try?"

"I'm game," said Race.

"Me, too," said Turk. "Let's go for it."

"Noon, then? We're free then. Good with you?" Marty asked Dave and Tony.

"Fine," said Tony, and Dave nodded.

It took three vets three hours of concentrated work to put that bobcat back together again. The leg bones were aligned and steel pins inserted to hold them in place. The entire hip joint had to be rebuilt. It was likely that the bobcat would limp, but if she healed, she would be walking, even running, on the rebuilt hip. Then the waiting began.

The recovering bobcat was put in the flight room. A wooden "A-frame" shelter went in one corner. Rugs and blankets formed a bed inside and the still-sleeping bobcat was gently placed inside.

"Now, it's up to you," said Dave. "Heal!" The odds had all been against her, but now she had a chance.

Dave remembered hearing similar words from a doctor when he was in the hospital after Vietnam. "Either you are a survivor, or you're not. It's up to you." He knew it was true. He had been determined to heal and to walk again, and despite all the cards stacked against him, he had come out a winner. He hoped for the same for the bobcat. He closed the flight room door.

The flight room is about fifteen by fifteen feet with a concrete floor and a drain in the middle for cleaning. A water faucet is in the wall, and attached to that is a hose with a steel nozzle so that the entire room can be hosed down. The bobcat's shelter was in the far right corner. In order to clean the room, it was necessary for two people to team up, one with a mop and the other with a broom. While the mop watched the bobcat, the broom swept, then the broom watched the bobcat while the mop mopped. When the room was basically clean, it was necessary to clean the bobcat area. Both mop and broom pushed the A-frame slowly to the opposite wall where fresh rugs and blankets made a new clean bed. The resident of the A-frame was reluctant to be out in the open and crept along with its slowly moving shelter, growling mightily at being disturbed. Finally, the A-frame reached the opposite wall, the bobcat had a clean bed, and the former bedding was thrown into the laundry and the corner cleaned. The next day the process was reversed.

This ritual went on reasonably comfortably until the day we

came in and found the hose uncoiled and stretched out all over the flight room. It was pretty obvious that the bobcat, a nocturnal animal, was ambulatory, and even feeling playful. After this, Dave had the volunteers place her food across the room from her shelter to make her move around and the hose was removed between cleanings to save it from destruction. Needless to say, after we knew the bobcat was mobile, extra precautions were taken when cleaning the flight room. This was one patient who was in no danger of being tamed! The Center staff adjusted.

After six weeks the cat had learned to walk around the flight room with the steel pins holding her bones securely. It was time to see how well the bones were healing. As Marty had said, cats heal quickly. The bobcat's radiographs were cause for rejoicing. The bones had knitted and all but one of the pins could be removed. The rebuilt hip was doing well. Dave and Tony started to think about release.

"Bill Meier said the farmer wanted her back in his territory. He said she'd be at home there," Tony reported after a phone call.

"I buy that," said Dave. "She'd have a better chance of survival if she were acquainted with her environment. She wouldn't have to find a new territory to defend. She would know where to hunt and where to drink. Good idea."

"I'll call Bob Baldwin. We want pictures for the newsletter." Tony started planning.

"How about the TV station? Think they would come?" asked Dave.

"No harm in trying. I'll call around," Tony agreed. "And the Times, of course. Dean will come. That bobcat will have a lot of media coverage when she takes off into the wild." Tony was grinning. A happy release was just the right sort of story to tell far and wide.

The bobcat cooperated by exercising her hind legs. She was young, a last year's kitten, and I thought she ought to have

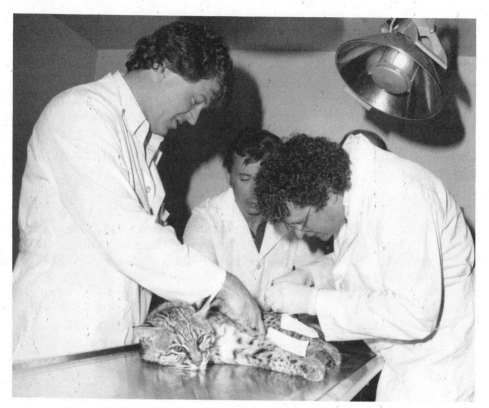

After several months of healing and bone-knitting, the bobcat's pins could be removed. The procedure was performed by Dr. Marty Smith, while Dr. Dave Theuerkauf and Dave Debauche held the cat.

something to play with since we had taken her hose away.

"Sybil, you're nuts!" Tony scoffed. "She's a wild animal. She wouldn't play with toys. Use your head."

"I know my cats," I insisted, "and she would, too, play with toys. She's just a youngster. I'll pick up something when I let the dogs out this noon. You just wait and see."

Every noon, I drove the seven miles home, let the dogs out, fixed a quick lunch and drove back to work. On this particular day, I stopped at the supermarket on my way back. In the pet department there was just the right ball for batting around the flight room, and just waiting for me was a catnip mouse. Just what I was looking for. I bought both and went back to the Center.

"I have the toys!" I called triumphantly as I came through the door. Tony came out of his office and Dave appeared from the back room.

"Are you serious?" asked Tony. "You really bought toys for that raving beast?"

"Don't tease. Yes, I bought the toys, and I am still betting she will play with them." I started unwrapping the ball and the mouse. "This is my contribution to her rehabilitation. If she does play with them, she will be running and jumping around and getting stronger and more ready to hunt. Isn't that worth a try?"

"All right. I give up," Tony said. "You win. Give her the toys."

"If it works, it's a plus. Worth a try," Dave agreed.

I opened the flight room door and threw in the ball. Not a move from the bobcat. Tony grinned. I threw in the mouse as close to a disinterested nose as I could. Surely the catnip would make a difference. Nothing. Tony put an arm around my shoulder.

"Good try," he consoled me, "but she's still a wild animal."

65

Dave shrugged. "It was still worth a try. She might have played with them. You never know. He returned to the back room and Tony and I went back to work in the front.

The next morning was R plus seven, just a week from the scheduled release. I unlocked the door and walked into my little corner. Then, out of curiosity, I walked toward the back and took a look into the flight room. Both the ball and the mouse were moved from where I had thrown them and both showed definite signs of wear and tear, mostly tear. A cat was a cat after all!

When Tony and Dave came in, I didn't say a word. I left it up to them. Would they notice?

"Hey, Sybil! Come here!" called Tony. "Dave, look at this! That crazy cat was playing last night! Look at those toys! I don't believe this!"

I walked to the flight room feeling smug. I bathed in their wonder and thoroughly enjoyed my one time in the rehabilitation sun. I don't know rehabilitation, but I do know my cats!

That day was when Tony and Dave decided to make catching the bobcat easier at the time of release. They went into the flight room and removed the A-frame, putting an animal carrier in the corner. When I asked why, Dave explained.

"If she accepts the carrier as her den instead of the A-frame, she will go into it when she is threatened. All we have to do is close the door. It beats tranquilizing her."

By this time, Warren had started his position as the new executive director of the Center. He and Tony were working together for the short time that Tony had left before going to Madison to register for summer classes. One of the first things he did was carry a tranquilized bobcat back from the Foster Smith Hospital to the Wildlife Center when the pins had been removed. He had not been around when the bobcat arrived, but he was definitely involved when the bobcat was released. It made a good start.

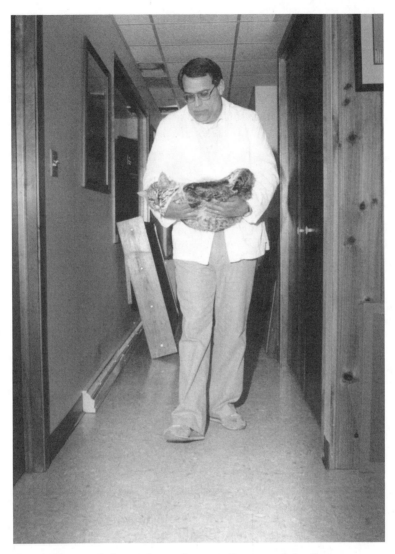

One of Warren's first jobs as the new director of the Center was to carry the bobcat back to the flight room after the pins had been removed.

Finally, the great day came. Bill Meier came to oversee the first part. Bob Baldwin came with his camera. The TV cameras were ready to film the capture of the bobcat in the flight room and to take pictures of the Center for background. Dean Bortz came from the *Lakeland Times,* and the heroine of the story behaved beautifully. When Dave and Tony entered the flight room (with a capture net, just in case), the bobcat retreated to her den, just as Dave had planned. He used the pole on the capture net to reach across and shut the carrier door. The bobcat was ready to go.

She did not, however, know the excitement which lay ahead of her. She spit and growled and snarled ferociously as her carrier was moved. All the cameras were humming and popping, which didn't help a bit — but we really did need the publicity. The cat had to endure.

Cat and cameras and her escorts were all loaded into various trucks and vans and the entourage headed for the farm between Tomahawk and Merrill. Roger and Joyce were waiting.

At about eleven, a parade of vehicles drove onto the farm. Bill Meier got out first. He was in charge.

"Hi!" he called. "Want your bobcat back?" He began to unhitch the tail gate to get at the carrier.

"How is he?" asked Joyce, approaching the truck. The cat yowled, and Joyce jumped back. "I guess he's all right," she laughed. "He certainly sounds healthy."

"It's a female, Joyce. Once we got her hindquarters out of the dirt and brush, it was pretty easy to tell 'he' was a she."

"Well, I'm glad she's back and whole again. We females have to stick together." Joyce smiled.

"Where are you going to release her? Where do we set up?" asked the cameraman from Channel 12.

Roger gestured down toward the woods along the edge of his fields. "Just beyond there the woods get thicker. He, er, she must have lived around there someplace and hunted in the open fields. It's kind of far down, but I don't want her all that close to the house."

"OK, Let's go." Bill Meier herded the group toward the woods. He and Dave were toting the carrier. The bobcat was not happy and let everyone know, in no uncertain terms.

"That's going to be something to hear in the middle of the night!" Bill told Roger. "You sure you want her back?"

"Sure as sure," Roger said. "This is where she belongs. Before she was hurt, we never knew she existed. I expect it will be that way again. We'll know she is out here somewhere, but we'll never see her, or hear her."

They trudged on. It was a cool spring day, but the sun was shining, and the smell of the earth in the fields was like a promise. Finally, they came to a deep ditch beyond the fields that ran into the woods and gradually widened and flattened out.

"This is a good place," said Bill. "Chances are she'll run along the ditch. If you want to set up here," he told the cameraman, "and let us know when you are ready, we'll open the door and let her run." He and Dave set the carrier on the edge of the ditch and waited while Bob Baldwin and the TV crew readied their equipment.

"I don't know about you guys," Bob Baldwin said, "but there's no way I am going to be in front of that carrier when they open the door!" He chose, instead, to set up his camera with the remote control. The camera would face the bobcat just in front of the carrier. The shutter would be controlled by a cautious man behind the carrier and out of harm's way. The TV crew focused ahead of the carrier, but the camera was safely behind it.

"Ready?" asked Bill Meier.

"I'm ready," said Bob Baldwin softly.

"Ready," said the TV man.

"OK, everybody? Here we go." Bill Meier opened the door of the carrier and stood back quickly.

Nothing happened.

Dave took a quick look at the front of the carrier. The bobcat's nose was up, and she was testing the air. It smelled familiar, but she had had so many bad experiences in the last few months that she wasn't even sure whether to trust her nose. She did not plan to move without being absolutely sure that the humans around her weren't going to spring another surprise on her. If she could just move fast enough...She gathered her now-strong back legs under her while behind the carrier everyone waited — and waited. Would the cat never go?

The TV cameraman sneaked a look at his watch and made a swift calculation as to how long he would have to get to his next assignment. Still the bobcat made no move.

Conscious of the impatience charging the air around him, Dave said to Bill Meier, "How about tipping the carrier a little?"

"Let's try it," Bill agreed.

The two men lifted the rear of the carrier a few inches off the ground. The bobcat dug her claws in and hung on tight. Sure enough, the humans had another surprise planned and she was sure she wouldn't like it. She continued to sit tight, albeit at a slight angle.

"Higher?" said Dave.

"Higher," nodded Bill Meier.

They raised the rear of the carrier up again. The cat sat tight.

"Nuts to this!" Bill Meier said. "Dump her out!" He and Dave lifted the back of the carrier almost to perpendicular and suddenly a tan blur shot out of the carrier, streaked down the ditch line and vanished, leaving open mouths behind it.

"Did you get it?" Dave asked the TV man.

"I have no idea. I think I got something, but I won't know until I get it developed. We can just hope. How about you?" he asked Bob Baldwin.

"Same here. I hope I got something. That cat was FAST!" Bob picked up his camera and checked it for possible damage.

Gradually, the crowd recovered and trekked back across the fields to the house.

"I made coffee," Joyce offered. "Anyone interested?"

The TV crew declined. Dean Bortz, from the *Times* had another assignment. Dave, Bill Meier, and Bob Baldwin joined Roger and Joyce in the spacious kitchen.

"It's been a long time," said Roger. "Tell you the truth, I didn't think she'd make it."

"Any other animal, she'd have been put down. Marty and the vets fixed her up because she was a cat. They heal fast," Dave explained.

"I'm glad she's back. I'm so glad you didn't shoot her." Joyce was looking directly at Bill Meier.

"Shoot her? Me? Joyce, are you crazy? Did you really think I would shoot her? I'm suppose to protect the wildlife in my area. You surprise me!"

"I'm sorry, Bill. All I could think of was that you would put her out of her misery. I was afraid shooting was the only answer."

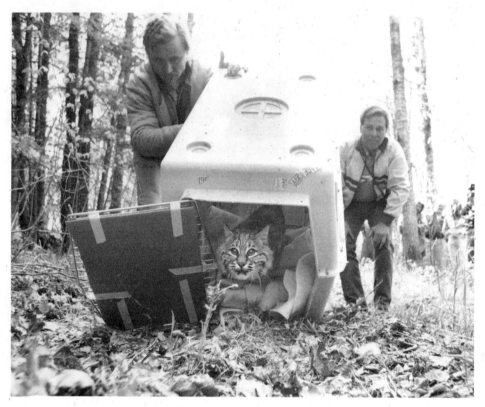

Tipping the reluctant bobcat toward freedom.

"It used to be," Bill Meier looked at Dave, "before there was a place to take them. Now we cart all the animals up to Dave and the vets at the hospital. You got any more coffee in the pot? I missed breakfast this morning."

The bobcat slowed down and stopped. No one was chasing her. She breathed heavily from her first hard run in several months. She looked around and felt comfortable with what she saw. She had not been here for a long time, but it was familiar. She turned and walked silently through the woods to a certain tree. She looked up to a certain branch. Her hip hurt slightly, but she was not to be deterred. She reached up and marked the tree trunk by scratching. This also pulled off some old nail sheaths. That had needed doing for a long time. With a bound she was four feet up the trunk. A few more efforts and she was sitting above the forest floor on an old familiar branch. She looked out across her territory. Satisfied, she stretched out on the branch and closed her eyes to contented slits. She was home.

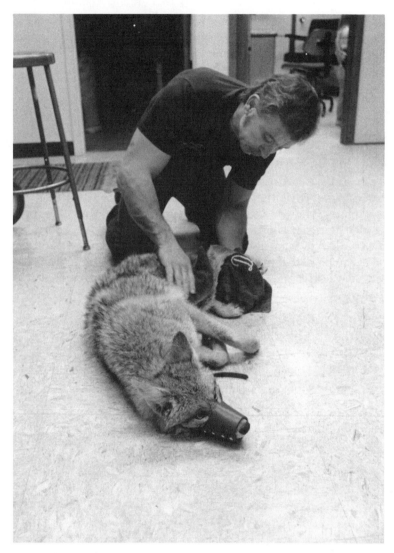

Dave cleans the paralyzed hindquarters of a female coyote, an auto accident victim.

A TALE OF A TAIL

The female coyote was brought in by the DNR. Because of the type of trauma, we assumed she was a car-strike victim. A spinal injury paralyzed her entire back end, inside and outside. She was unable to move her hind legs or tail, and unable to control either bowel or bladder. The front end, however, was in great shape, and that, unfortunately, is the business end of a coyote. Imagine trying to take a nice warm wet wash cloth and clean up the back end while the front end is slashing at you with a complete set of super sharp teeth! And believe me, she took a LOT of cleaning up!

As you might guess, it was a two-person job. Occasionally I was commandeered for the job. Never, never say that I volunteered. I was desperately sorry for her, and would have felt more comfortable on the clean-up detail, messy as it was, in preference to the job I was given: to control the front part with a "catch pole."

First, Dave opened the cage. Despite the fact that we both knew she wasn't going any place, she LOOKED as if she would bound out chomping at anything in the way. She HAD to look ferocious, poor thing, because she knew that she was cornered by her own body. All she could do was fight. She certainly couldn't run to safety.

The next step was to open the loop on the catch-pole and slip it over her head. Naturally, she fought every effort. As the noose came close she snapped at it. If I caught a tiny bit of muzzle, the proud head would shake itself free. Remember, I am maneuvering outside the cage at the end of a long pole. What control I had was the back and forth motion of a slip handle which enlarged and shortened the wire. The pole was about the length of a broom stick, which is reassuring when you have finally caught your animal and can keep it that far away, but it makes for a very difficult catch. It's like threading a sewing machine needle at arm's length while the machine is operating. At last, I was able to slip her whole head into the loop simply because Dave, bless his heart, distracted her for me. Quickly, I closed the noose and held her head while Dave gently eased her out of the dirty cage and onto the treatment room floor. She smelled terrible, and must have hated it. Animals are naturally clean, and do not soil themselves or their bedding.

Dave cleaned her up while she struggled to get free of the noose. I had to hold her tightly enough to keep Dave's hands safe, but loosely enough not to strangle her. It's a neat trick!

I always expect a wild animal to realize that we are trying to help it, and to cooperate in the effort. This is sheer hogwash and only proves how much I don't know. The only thing an animal has on its mind is to get away from these humans as fast as possible, by any means within its power.

Several times daily, the coyote had to suffer the indignity of having her private parts washed and dried while a horrible human held her head. You would think she would feel so much better, lying clean and fresh on clean bedding, that eventually she would get the idea that the process resulted in a good feeling and should be endured more stoically. Not at all. Every day she fought, but one day, a back leg moved! The swelling in the spinal cord was going down and the nerves were able once again to send their messages to her leg. It began to look as if all the care was worth the effort.

Slowly, she regained the use of her legs. This made the clean-up job more difficult, but it was still necessary, as she had not yet regained bowel or bladder control, nor could she move her tail. We waited. And waited.

She ate well. All vital signs were A-OK. She was even gaining weight. No, we did not weigh her, but her skinny ribs were now covered, and her coat was in good condition. All she needed was to regain control. We still waited.

One week went by, two weeks, three. She stood now, but the waste oozed out of her. She did not squat, nor was she able to move her tail out of the way. She was still a smelly, dirty mess.

"This isn't going to work," Dave said finally. "It looks like she's come as far as she's going to." He sighed as he directed her back into her cage with the catch-pole.

"But she's walking!" I cried. Obviously, she was. Dave released the noose and closed the cage door.

"But she has no control, and she can't move her tail. I can't release her like that!" Dave spoke angrily, which meant he was thoroughly frustrated and upset.

"Can't we wait a little longer?" I begged.

"Think!" he said grimly. "She's a pack animal! What's a pack going to do with her? Think of the flies! They'd drive her crazy! All that dirt will cause sores and infection! And her tail! That's how they communicate! It's up. It's down! It wags! That's how they talk! And she can't even wag her tail!" He banged on the counter and stalked around the room as he talked. "OK! One week. I'll give her one more week! But I'm telling you it won't do any good. Her spine healed, but the nerves didn't all come back. It happens." He grabbed the trash bag and tied the corners together. Yanking it out of the waste paper basket, he headed for the dumpster. "One more week! That's all!" He banged out the door, miserable and frustrated.

It was an awful week of waiting. That tail became a CAUSE! Day after day it hung limp and useless. Not a quiver. Every day she was filthy and needed cleaning. If ever a wild animal had humans pulling for it, that coyote was it. All three vets examined her and tested reflexes. Nothing. The volunteers checked her several times a day. Nothing. Even the secretary walked into the back room to check a tail. It was still limp and useless. The week passed.

Saturday morning, when I came in, Marty and Turk were walking out of the back room. They said good morning, but without the usual banter and teasing. Something was up. I started down the hall to the back room, but I saw Dave coming out of the storage room with the spade. It was over. I stopped and turned back. I didn't want to know. I didn't want to see. There was a big lump in my throat. It was a long time before I could see clearly enough to work. If only she could have wagged her tail!

GRILLED OWL

A summer resident was driving north from Chicago to his cottage in the Minocqua area. Just beyond Wausau, a huge bird flew in front of the car. The driver jammed on the brakes, sure he had hit the bird. His headlights picked up nothing that might have been thrown in front of the car at the impact. He pulled off the road and walked back along the shoulder. No bird. He went back and got his flashlight and searched the ditch. No bird. He shook his head, climbed back into his car and drove on to Minocqua.

When he arrived, he and his friend unpacked the trunk and went into the cottage. The two men spent the early evening turning on the electricity, priming the pump, which refused to run after a winter's rest, and picking up all the empty mouse traps that were supposed to have caught unwelcome winter guests. They ate the sandwiches they had brought, washing them down with pop from a cooler, as the refrigerator was still warm. They walked around outside, planning to put in the dock the following day and get the boat in the water for fishing. Eventually, they made their beds and called it a day.

The next morning it was necessary to stock up at the grocery store. Their wives and children were to arrive today, and they had promised to open the cottage and have everything ready. Off to the store they went. For the first time, they walked around the front of the car.

"Son-of-a-gun! Look at this!" said the friend, as he walked around from the passenger side.

"What's up?" asked the driver, as he closed his door.

"Remember the bird you couldn't find last night?" the friend said pointing to the front of the car. "Here he is!"

The driver stared incredulously. "I never thought to look at the grill!"

There, securely stuck, was a large barred owl plastered up against the grill of the car.

The two men looked in wonder. Then, assuming it was dead, they went into the store and did their shopping. After they had unloaded everything at the cottage, the man who had been driving spoke. "I'd better get that carcass out of the car before the kids come."

"I'll help. How are you going to do it? You'll have to pick it out one piece at a time."

The driver picked up a screw driver from the utility drawer. "I may have to undo the whole grill." The two men went outside. When they got around to the front of the car, the bird opened its eyes.

"It's alive! That crazy son-of-a-gun is alive! Can you believe it?" exclaimed the friend.

"How can he be alive? I must have hit him hard. Then he was stuck there all the way when we were driving, and all last night! This is unbelievable!"

"Now what are you going to do?" asked the friend. "That's a big bird!"

"I'm not going to do anything. The Wildlife Center is. I know the man who runs it. I'll give him a call."

Warren took the call. Chuckling, he turned from the phone when he had hung up. "We've got a grilled bird to pick up. From what he says, it's an owl. Who wants to go?"

All the interns were there at the time, plus the back room volunteer. Naturally everyone wanted to go. But the truck only held three at the most. "I'll take my car," said Hadie, and in a few minutes, I was the only one at the Center.

They were gone about an hour, returning with the sorriest

looking barred owl I have ever seen. He had obviously been through a lot. Not a feather was in place, and his head hung limp. "Is he alive?" I asked Dave.

"Just barely," he answered and disappeared into the back room. He started fluids immediately, giving it electrolytes and treating it for shock. Having administered what first aid he could, Dave put it in a cage where it lay inert. It's chances looked pretty slim.

Dave let it recover for a while, and administered more fluids. The bird just lay on the bottom of the cage, eyes closed. Dave kept him quiet and put a cloth over the cage door to darken it. Nothing to do but wait.

The next day, the owl was still alive. But he was still not perching. There is nothing so discouraging to a rehabilitator as a bird who cannot or will not perch. Dave sighed. More fluids. Later in the day, Dave force-fed the bird an ounce of mouse, and later another ounce. Still the doggone owl lay on the cage bottom. An X-ray showed a broken clavicle. This was taped in place, but still the bird lay on the bottom of the cage and had to be force fed. Not good.

Finally, after an agonizing week of worry and care, Dave came in one morning to find the grilled owl sitting on his perch and trying to peck off the tape on his shoulder.

"Hey. Look at you! Look at this, everybody! Look who's perching!" Dave called happily, and we all cheered and patted Dave on the back. From then on the owl recovered rapidly. Then it was time to take off the tape and put the bird in an outside flight cage to exercise. He did well. He ate voraciously. Finally, it was time to fly him on a creance.

A creance (kree-ons) is like a fishing reel with heavy line, and a short handle. Jesses (jess-ez), or leather straps, are put on the bird's ankles, and the long creance line is attached to the jesses. The bird is taken to an open space and allowed to fly to the end of the creance. Then he is able to fly around and around, while the rehabilitator watches the flight to see that the wings are used evenly and strongly. When the bird becomes tired, it is reeled in like a fish on a line, caught, and taken back to its cage till the next exercise session. In this way, a bird which has been immobilized by a broken wing, or in the grilled owl's case, a broken shoulder, has an opportunity to regain his muscle tone before he is released into the wild.

The grilled owl did very well, and a few days later, two of the interns who had been in the crowd who picked him up had the honor of releasing him. He was not released in the Wausau area where he came from, but you might see him in the woods around Minocqua.

ONE INJURED FAWN

The doe strained one more time and the tiny fawn was born. The doe turned and licked it clean, not realizing that the stimulation of her rough tongue helped the fawn's first breath, and cleaned its nostrils. After taking care of the baby's first moments, it was time to feed him. The tired doe stood up and nudged her fawn. Coordination was not his highest skill at this age, and he had trouble getting his long legs to follow his will. They went in every direction except under him. He fell back a number of times. Then he got lucky, and everything worked at once. At last! He was on his feet, staggering a little, it's true, but upright at last!

He shuffled around and found his mother's teat. These next few meals were his most important. The colostrum, which he would get before the milk supply was established, protected him against disease and infection. Without it, he could quickly become sick and die.

After he had eaten, both the doe and the fawn lay together, resting in an area a little withdrawn from the birth area. Instinctively, the doe knew that her scent there was strong and would attract predators. It was best to move away. After a rest, the doe stood up and left her fawn still sleeping. She would browse for a while and drink before she returned to feed him again. The fawn slept on.

The next time she fed her baby, the doe made him stand and leave the place where she had been feeding him. She nudged him with her nose until he had moved several yards away. He found a grassy spot in a field, stood swaying for a while, and lay down again. He was still very new. But instinct would protect him. Satisfied that he was safe, the doe again left.

A fawn, for the first few wobbly days, has no scent. The little buck fawn would be perfectly safe from predators if he lay still and made no sound. Predators are scent hunters. If they can't smell it, it isn't there. A coyote could walk right past our little fawn,

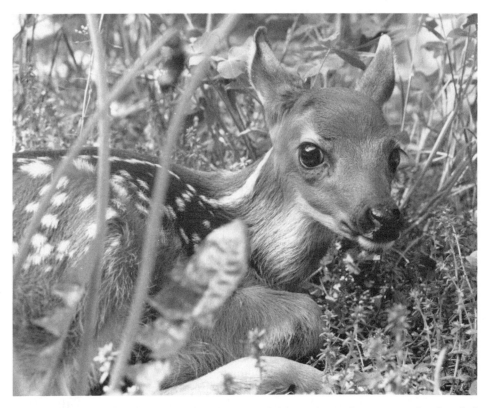

A week-old whitetail deer fawn lies silent and motionless where its mother has left it, while she browses for food nearby.

even sight it, but if his nose didn't "see" it, it wasn't there. An analogy to human experience is our dependence on the sense of touch. When we say, "Let me see it," we are at the same time, reaching out a hand to hold it and touch it. When Hamlet sees the dagger and cannot clutch it, he decides it is a "dagger of the mind" and does not exist. If we can't feel it, it isn't there.

Instinctively knowing this, the fawn lay still. The doe, who had a scent, stayed away from him except for feeding, after which she made the baby move away again.

When his mother left one time, both he and she were uneasy. There was a big noise in the distance. It was not a forest noise, and was not to be trusted. The doe stood off in the forest near the tall grass where her fawn lay. She browsed, but she watched. The noise was coming closer. There was a cloud of dust coming across the grass and the dust was making a huge racket. She wanted to run, but she was worried. She moved back into the forest, but turned to watch the cloud. It was getting close to her fawn. The noise was louder. The doe was trembling.

The fawn was terrified of the big noise, but lay still. Not an ear twitched, but both eyes were wide open with fear. The noise and the cloud were coming closer. Suddenly, the doe turned, put up her white tail as a flag, and bounded into the woods. Seeing his mother's signal, just as the cloud was on him, he gathered his long legs and made a jump after her. He was not fast enough, the cloud bit his back leg. He called for his mother in pain. His tiny voice sounded like the bleat of a lamb. The doe stopped in mid-bound and turned. The noise stopped. The cloud dissipated, and the farmer who had been cutting in that field jumped down off his machine and ran to the injured fawn. As the doe watched helplessly, the farmer picked up the bleating fawn, and putting him on his lap, started the combine again and headed for the farmhouse.

When he got to the farmyard, he gently placed the bleeding fawn in an unused dog run, and hurried inside for bandaging materials. When he had bound the bleeding leg sufficiently to enable the fawn to travel in the truck, the farmer took him to the vet.

"I can't save the hoof," the doctor said after examining the little buck. "He'll probably heal up and form a callous on the stump, but I can't put him back together."

"What'll I do with him?" the farmer asked. "Poor little guy. I never saw him till it was too late." He stroked the tiny spotted body. "Something like this makes a fellow feel real bad."

"You could try the Wildlife Center down in Minocqua. They take care of wild animals. They'd probably take him or find a place for him. I'll give them a call, OK?"

The farmer nodded.

That is when the call came in from the Ashland veterinarian about the fawn with the amputated hoof as a result of a farm accident. The call came at a time when the Center was something of a madhouse. There were two programs scheduled back to back: one a school group on its end-of-semester trip, and right after them a busload of senior citizens were coming as part of an Elderhostel trip. The back room was buzzing with baby animal feedings, and so guess who got the job of being an animal ambulance for the fawn? Right.

I drove north on Highway 51 on a beautiful spring day, feeling guilty about escaping from the Center chaos. The farm was on this side of Ashland, and I was able to find it easily.

"Hi! I'm from the Wildlife Center. Here to pick up a fawn?" I turned my statement into a question, because there was no fawn in sight.

"Right here. Just a minute," said the big, burly man who had come out to greet me.

I got out of the car and opened the back. I had brought a dog carrier, and had loaded the bottom with pads and a blanket. The farmer soon reappeared out of a dog pen with the fawn in his arms. A big golden retriever came out with him, tail wagging, and a big "smile" on his face. The two animals had apparently

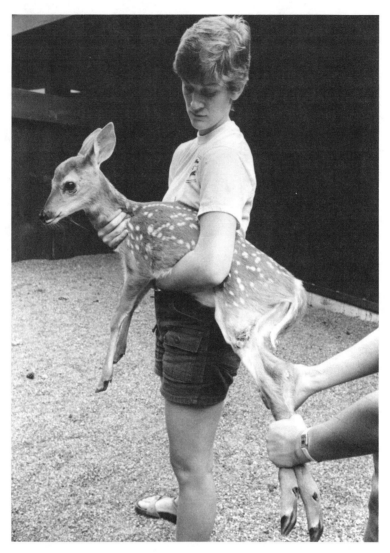

Kathy Snell, a veterinary student intern, holds an injured fawn.

been housed together and had gotten along famously. The farmer slipped the little fawn into the dog pen in the car and closed the door. He stood there a minute looking at the little buck.

"I think I just quit hunting," he said ruefully. He sighed a deep sigh, and backed away from the car.

"Thank you very much!" I said, as I got in the car. "We'll take good care of him."

The farmer waved briefly as I drove off.

Marty looked over the fawn's hoof when he arrived, but the Ashland vet had done a super job and no further work was necessary. Time and the fawn's youth would be the healers now. The fawn went into the courtyard and was fed from a bottle, which he didn't approve of at all. Eventually, he accepted this odd method of eating and spent the summer growing and healing, although he did not grow as large as he might have if he had had the advantage of his mother's milk. Doe milk is very rich, and so far, no one has come up with a satisfactory replacement for orphaned fawns.

In the fall, he was released at Dairyman's Country Club, a private club north of Minocqua where the deer are fed all winter, and where hunting is not allowed. Our little fawn would be well cared for, and would become a member of the resident herd.

The doe had stood in the forest and watched her fawn being carried away. She waited, but he did not return. She went into the field where the noise and the cloud had been. Her sensitive nose smelled his blood on the earth. She pawed at the place. She looked all around and risked calling him. Her voice, too, sounded like the bleat of a lamb. There was no answer. She stood quietly a moment looking down. Slowly, she went back into the forest.

SOME FLIGHT ROOM INMATES

Right now, the flight room contains four offices. Warren, the director, Dave and Jacquie, the rehabilitators, and I, the secretary, all share space in the room. It's been this way for about a year, and in another year all the offices will be elsewhere and the flight room will become the baby animal nursery.

Originally, the flight room was intended for birds needing to practice flying under safe indoor conditions. Baby birds would learn to fly. Injured birds which had been caged for a long time with broken bones would exercise in the flight room and regain their muscle tone. Often, it was used for that purpose.

Five baby barred owls learned to fly and to catch their prey in the flight room. Seven little kestrels also learned flying and hunting here. If you stop to think, for a small bird of prey, just learning to fly is not enough. If they are to survive, they have to develop their hunting skills. They may be born with the hunting instinct, but are far from being good at it. To send a small, inexperienced hunter out into the wild is to send him to his death by starvation. He needs some learning experience.

How does he get it? Before I answer that question, let me explain that in nature it is eat or be eaten. There are predators and there are prey animals. Most predators have eyes in the front of their heads, and have binocular vision just as you do. Most prey animals have eyes on the sides of their heads which function independently and enable the prey animal to see both sides at once as he watches for danger. First, think of the owl, the hawk, the coyote, the bobcat. All these are predators. Now think of the mouse, the squirrel, the rabbit, and the robin. These are all prey animals. The former is destined by nature to eat the latter. What may seem cruel to humans is simply the way life is in the wild.

In our flight room, to teach the baby predators to hunt, whether they are mammals or birds, we release prey animals into the flight room and watch to be sure each baby predator is able to catch its dinner with enough skill to do it in the wild.

When it was time for the baby barred owls to learn, Mark first tied a dead laboratory mouse on a line and threw it in the flight room door. With the line he caused it to "run" across the room. All little owl eyes were on it. Although they are primarily auditory hunters, no owl will ignore prey dragged right in front of its vision. Nobody pounced. They just watched this odd thing going from one place to another. Mark finally gave up and decided to let them practice on the real thing.

The next day, they were not given their freshly thawed dead mice. Instead five live mice were released into the room. Naturally, the first thing the mice did was hide behind the tree stumps. Every now and then a mouse would decide there must be a better hiding place and would change tree stumps. The baby owls watched. Nothing happened. It was after four and the people went home.

The next morning the mice were gone. Who ate them? That was easy! Whoever ate would spit up a pellet of mouse hair and bones that he was unable to digest! The owls had favorite perching spots, and pellets in that general vicinity meant the percher at that spot had eaten. Since there were five pellets properly distributed, it could be assumed that the five baby owls had consumed the five mice. Easy!

When the process was again successfully completed, the babies were considered skilled enough hunters to try it in the wild. Out came the hacking box. It was placed on top of the high school football field's broadcasting booth. The owls hunted at night, and food was put in the box in the morning for anyone who didn't make a kill. In two days, that was no longer necessary. The baby owls had gone their own ways. The hacking box was removed. The owls' chart was marked "Released."

Mammals, too, had to learn by doing. One baby red fox who had been hit by a car and had recently recovered from a broken rear leg was given an opportunity to sharpen his hunting skills, and test the mended leg before release. A chipmunk was live-trapped for him. The chipmunk scurried for his life with the young fox bouncing behind him. The chipmunk ran up one of the stumps and jumped down the other side. The little fox jumped up on the stump and down after him, but the chipmunk had done him in. The jump broke the fox's front leg and back he went into a cast and a small cage again. The winning chipmunk was released!

Another resident of the flight room was a pileated woodpecker. This crow-sized woodpecker is the one you see in the cartoons. "Woody Woodpecker" is a pileated woodpecker with his red-crested head. He is easily identifiable because of his huge size, but he is rarely seen because he chooses lonely areas where there are few houses and people, and is a master at hiding on the OTHER side of a tree. Often evidence of the big pileated is easier to find than the bird himself. He pecks huge rectangular holes in dead trees and the chips from those holes are correspondingly huge. Remember this.

Our woodpecker had a broken wing from a car strike and was taped up and held in a small cage until healing had gone far enough along to enable him to be placed in the flight room where he had more room to match his size. MISTAKE!

The woodpecker literally demolished the room! He pecked the stumps until they were a pile of chips. Since both stumps had once been substantial trees and had been cut to fit the flight room from floor to ceiling, complete with several branches each for perching, that was some pecking job! The bird then moved on to better things. He decided the walls were just one big tree and proceeded to batter them down as well. It seemed not to matter to him that they were drywall and not wood. He pecked happily away. We couldn't wait until his wing was sufficiently healed for the pins to be removed and for him to be OUT of the flight room. The continual rat-tat-tat-tat was unnerving when you knew that it was walls he was demolishing!

Finally the great day came. The pins were removed. At last we could put him in an outside flight cage. We swept up the latest piles of plaster, and Dave started working with patching plaster and paint. New trees had to be measured and cut for the next inhabitants, and finally the flight room was usable again. The woodpecker had now regained his muscle tone and was taken back to the remote woodlands he had come from and released. Good-bye, and this time, good riddance!

"BUCK-DOGGING"

The hero of this story was not technically one of our patients. He was a young deer who had been raised by the Department of Natural Resources. He was in an enclosure behind the courthouse in Crandon. Despite care, one day he managed to get his new antlers entangled in the wire fence and the more he fought the fence, the more wire pulled out and wove itself in and amongst the branches of his antlers until he wore a wire crown and was frantic with fear and frustration.

The phone rang at the Center.

"Northwoods Wildlife Center. This is Sybil. May I help you?"

"Hi! Sybil. This is Ron at the Crandon Ranger Station. We have a deer all tangled up in fencing. Is Dave around?"

"Sure. Just a minute." I covered the phone and hollered into the back room. "Dave!"

Dave picked up the phone and listened. A few minutes later he appeared at the front desk armed with a set of wire cutters. At that moment Bob Baldwin walked through the door. He looked at Dave and his artillery.

"What's up?"

Dave explained and invited Bob to go with him. Never one to pass up a photo opportunity, Bob accepted with alacrity and the two of them vanished into the truck.

An hour later they reached the county courthouse preserve. Ron was at the front entrance to meet them.

"Wow! Am I glad to see you! That poor buck has just about had it. Nobody dares get near him. He's wild!"

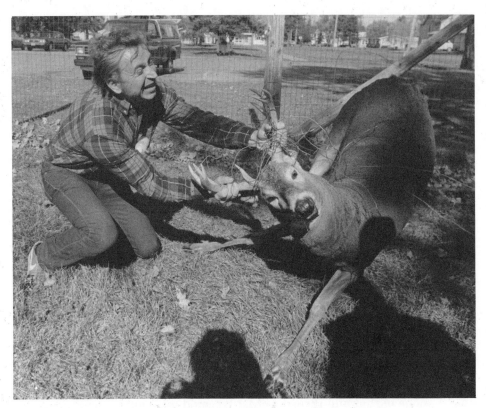

The precise moment when Dave's thumb was broken in his wrestle with the wired deer. The visible shadows are those of Dave's transfixed helpers.

"That's reassuring," Dave said mildly. "I've got the clippers. How many guys do you have to help?"

"Five, counting me," Ron answered. "Come over this way."

He walked down a path toward the back of the public building. Farther to the back was an enclosure containing a small cyclone. The buck, crowned with wire, was snorting, pawing and blowing. By now, his head was nearly immobilized. He was terrified. A small group of men were standing well away from the enclosure discussing how best to solve their problem. They were visibly relieved to see Dave.

Dave stopped and surveyed the situation. It wasn't going to be easy. Deer, which look so calm and placid when browsing through the woods, are tough fighters. Not only do they use their antlers, which in this instance were pretty well taken care of, but their sharp hooves are formidable weapons. One well-placed hoof can lay open cheek, chest and belly in an instant, and is nothing to treat lightly.

Dave opened his small case and prepared a tranquilizer shot. The problem, of course, was to get it in the deer. First, he tried the obvious, and approached from the rear. The deer would have none of that and turned as best he could to keep his enemy in front of him. After a few futile tries at this strange dance, Dave called a halt.

"I'll have to take him down," he said. "All of you watch, and when I get him down, you all come in and sit on him. Grab a leg, four of you, and keep him down. I'll turn him loose and poke the shot in. Right?"

"Right!" Heads nodded, and a general murmur indicated that the positions were being decided. Dave crawled slowly through the hole in the fence. The deer turned to face him. Dave maneuvered for position like a wrestler in the ring, hands at the ready, poised to spring. At just the right moment, he jumped, grabbed the antlers and twisted the neck until the deer fell to its knees like a calf at a rodeo. But he didn't go down without putting up a valiant and spectacular battle with his oppressor. When Dave finally got him down, he looked up to alert his helpers. To a man, they were plastered at the fence with pained expressions on their faces and clutching the wire for dear life! They had unconsciously adopted Dave's expression and had so completely empathized into his struggles with the deer that they were immobilized momentarily. When Dave looked up, he broke the spell. Still no one moved. In desperation, he threw a leg over the front quarters of the buck, and holding the antlers tight to the ground with one hand and arm, he extricated the tranquilizer needle from his back pocket. Just as he was about to use his teeth to remove the safety cover Ron shouted.

"Wait! No! Don't tranquilize him! The last deer we tranquilized died! Just clip the wire!"

Dave stared at him incredulously. Now, however, was no time to argue.

The buck was breathing heavily and would soon make another effort at escape. He returned the needle to his pocket, this time removing the wire clippers. By now, Bob Baldwin had put down his camera and was holding the bucks rear quarters. Dave began cutting wires. The other helpers descended on the buck and sat on him to hold him quiet. Dave clipped as fast as he could one-handed, first cutting the wires which bound the buck to the fence. He then clipped away at the entangled antlers, always keeping the deer's head and forequarters tight to the ground. He was, in effect, sitting astride the buck.

When the antlers were freed from the wire, he told his assistants to get to safety. Dave then had the difficult problem of relieving the pressure on the buck's head and shoulders and getting safely away before he was gored by an antler or disemboweled by a hoof. His own physical problems made it difficult to move with any agility. With his bad back, his bad leg, and his scarred arms, he had to find a way through the fence. The hole, however, was on the other side of the deer. There was no way he could beat the buck to the opening. He then decided that the deer was just as anxious to get away from his tormentor as he, Dave, was to get

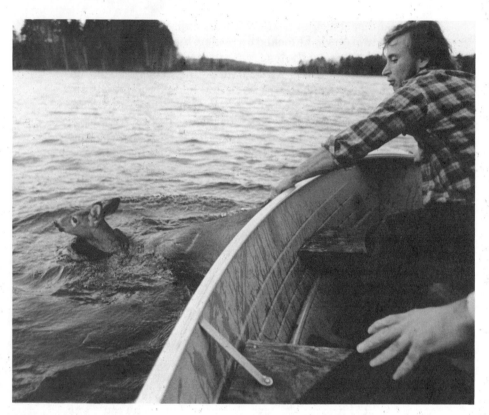

This whitetail doe was hit by a car on a bridge, thrown right through the railing and into the water. Dave was able to rescue the doe, but she was so badly injured that she had to be euthanized.

away from the deer. In one quick move, he released both antlers and forequarters and rolled away from the deer. He had guessed right. The frantic buck jumped up and vaulted through the fence opening into the open fields and then stopped, shaking his head as if he couldn't believe what had happened. Dave picked himself up from the ground and took physical inventory as he brushed himself off. He knew he'd be sore for days afterwards, but aside from a very painful sprained thumb, he had escaped without injury.

The buck, no doubt, would have a sore neck from being wrestled to the ground, but at least he was free.

"I got some great pictures!" said Bob Baldwin as Dave left the enclosure. "You should have seen the expression on your face!"

"Nice job," said Ron. "Thanks a lot. Don't know how we could have done it without you."

Dave grinned his famous grin. He and Bob climbed into the truck.

"All in a day's work," said Dave as they drove back to the Center.

"What happened to the deer they were talking about?" Bob asked. "The one that died."

"They tranquilized it to bring it up to the Center. It had been shot in the bow season. Had a bad sore on the flank. Infected. Somehow it got its head twisted around in the crate and suffocated. It was dead when they got to the Center. They blamed the tranquilizer." Dave drove silently for a while. Then he spoke. "It's funny, you do the best you can for an animal. Sometimes it's not good enough."

"You did a heck of a job today, though," Bob chuckled. "You should have seen your face."

RACCOON BABIES

There is nothing more appealing than a baby raccoon. Of all the wildlife babies, the raccoons with their little bright eyes and masked faces seem to melt more hearts and end up as someone's pets more than any other wild animals. When they get big enough to pose some danger to the family's baby, or the family dog or cat, the baby raccoons are brought to the Center to be rusticated. We do the best we can, but we'd much rather have orphans BEFORE anyone else has had a chance to pet and baby them and get them accustomed to man. Wild animals need to be wild.

We do not go so far as some centers do, and deliberately, by kicking the cages, yelling loudly, and making sudden loud noises, keeping them terrified of what awful humans are going to do next. We simply handle them as little as possible, keep them clean and cared for, but basically left alone. We wean them onto natural foods and let them go where the habitat is right for them. Instinct has to take over. At least they will not head for the nearest house.

Caring for raccoons, both young and older, can be dangerous to the ignorant caretaker. Some raccoons carry an intestinal parasite which is of no particular danger to the raccoon, but could be a serious danger to an unsuspecting human who is not warned about scrupulous cleanliness. Cleaning cages is the biggest problem, since cage cleaners are removing the feces and washing down the cages. If the caretaker does not scrub up his own hands afterwards, he runs into the possibility of infecting himself with the parasite. However, what is an intestinal parasite in raccoons becomes a brain parasite in humans. Instead of multiplying in an intestine where it can be expelled, it multiplies in the brain and eventually kills its host.

People who take in a family of baby raccoons because they are "so cute" should be advised to be very careful. Much better to bring the animal family to a wildlife center which is prepared to give them proper care under strict rules of cleanliness for the caretakers. This includes the use of rubber gloves which are discarded after use. Needless to say, all raccoons are not infested, but all should be treated as if they were.

Last summer, we were brought a family of four raccoon babies which had been home-raised and loved. They were hand-fed dainties from the table, they lap-sat in the evenings and were treated like kittens might be. We were to try to return them to the wild. Not easy.

For a few weeks, we kept them at the Center, giving them the "leave them alone" treatment. They had each other, but they did not have human company. Then it was time to hack them out. "Hacking" is a technique used primarily with releasing birds. The bird babies are placed in a box in a tree where they are free to come and go as they feel comfortable. Food is placed in the box daily. If a small owl or hawk can catch his own dinner, he'd rather have that, but if he can't, he can always return to the hacking box for a handout until his hunting skills are honed. We thought there was no reason not to try the same technique on the small raccoons.

Because I live in the woods near a marsh LOADED with frogs and other raccoon goodies, my property was chosen for the release. Besides, I was always around to check up on their food. Jacquie Quesnell, now our rehabilitator with Dave, was at that time an intern from the University of Wisconsin School of Veterinary Medicine. She put the four raccoons in carriers, and we put the carriers in the back of my car. Off to the woods.

While Jacquie unloaded the animals, I dug a hole in the ground and put a wooden box on top to make a den. Inside the hole I placed a small pile of the food they had been eating at the Center and which I would continue to make available for them. Jacquie and I carried the carriers to the "den" and released the babies. Curious to a fault, they examined everything. In and out of the den they crawled. Up on the box they climbed. They made small excursions into the blackberry brambles behind the "den" which would mean safety if they needed it.

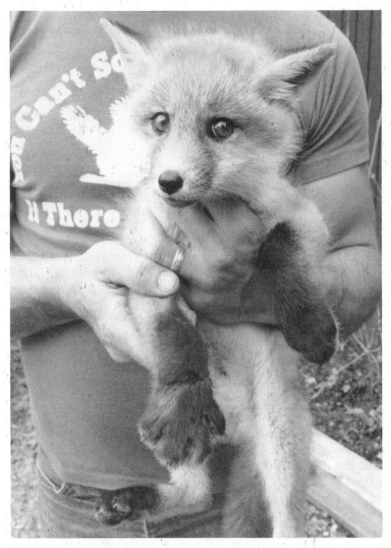

The front paw of a baby fox shows signs of injury by a steel jaw trap, a common hazard to northwoods wildlife.

Satisfied that we had done the best we could, Jacquie and I started back to the car.

"Whoops!" exclaimed Jacquie, as she nearly stumbled over all four raccoons who were practically walking between her legs in their anxiety not to be left behind.

"What do we do now?" she asked.

"I don't know. Just escape the best we can. If you will walk them back to the 'den', I will get the car started and leave the door open. Then run like the dickens," I suggested. It wasn't going to be easy.

It wasn't. Four raccoons determined not to be abandoned can run like the dickens, too. It took several tries, but we finally left four forlorn raccoon babies watching the car escape down the road without them.

When I came home about four-thirty there were no raccoons in sight. Good. They had probably taken off into the woods. I let my dogs out into their yard. The dogs are basset hounds and the yard is fenced and large enough for twenty-one trees and plenty of running around room which my son, Bill, keeps cut with the lawnmower, although I cannot dignify the area by calling it grass. It is simply a chunk of fenced-in woods. By the time I had my office clothes off and my home clothes on, the dogs were barking wildly, and I went outside. There were the four raccoons — two sitting on trees just outside the fence and two teetering on the fence itself. I went out and grabbed a couple of dog collars and brought the owners into the house.....followed by the two fence raccoons who planned to come in, too. My basset hounds are the world's mellowest dogs, but invasion by raccoon strangers is not to be borne. They continued to bark and tried to engage the intruders in combat. I was using both feet and both hands to keep the animals separate, and to throw determined raccoons out the door and get it closed before they could pop in again. I finally made it only to have one baby spread-eagled on the screen trying to come in the window. By this time the cats were involved and climbing the screens, too. I peeled the cats off the inside and

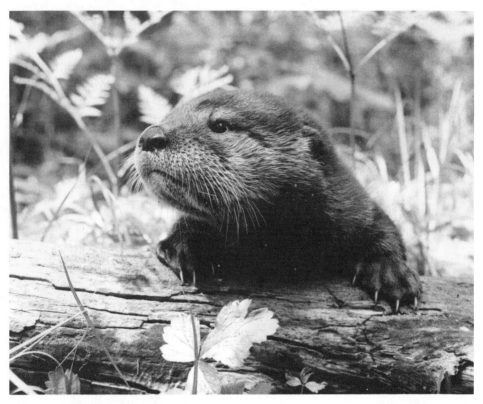

This orphaned baby otter was brought to the Center by forest service workers in the Nicolet National Forest.

closed the window. The raccoon gave up and dropped off.

All night, pitiful little cries came from unhappy raccoon babies who wanted to join the inside group. My impulse was to go out and cuddle them happy, but I knew better and hardened my heart against those sad little cries.

The next morning, two met me as I fed the birds and put fresh food in the hacking box "den." I managed to sneak back into the house without incident, but had a problem going to work since they followed me into the garage and I had to get them out before I could close the garage door.

That evening, when I got home, no raccoons! The dogs went out and came in. No raccoons. I figured the two who had been on the tree were adapting to the wild, and now, it seemed that the two who followed the dogs in were also deciding to make it on their own. What a relief!

But the phone rang a couple of hours later.

"This is Bonnie Passow. I'm your new neighbor down the hill. I know you work for the Wildlife Center. Do you know anything about raccoons?"

My heart sank. "How many?" I asked.

"Well, two baby raccoons are hanging around the house and I'm afraid something will happen to them. They are so tame. They want to come in the house."

"Don't let them in or you'll never get them out. I'll be right down and pick them up." I put my shoes back on and got the dog carrier into the car and drove down the hill to Passow's. There was Bonnie, out on her patio in a lounge chair with the two babies on her lap.

"Can you believe this?" she said. "Look how tame they are!"

"I believe it," I said, and picked them up and put them in the

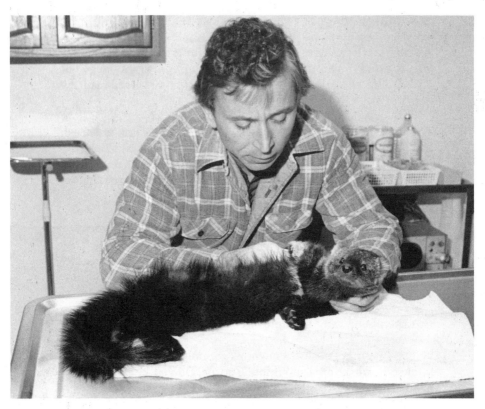

Dave examines a fisher that has sustained injuries from a trap.

carrier. "Thank you so much for calling me." We talked a while, and I drove back home. I put food in the carrier and kept the babies in it all night. Back to the Center they went the next day.

What to do? Warren, who was now the director, called a wildlife lover he knew who lived in a really wild area on a remote lake shore where other raccoons made their home. He asked whether it would be all right if we rusticated the two babies on his property. Warren would come by daily with the food for hacking. The man agreed, and once again, the babies were transported to a new home. This time, after the first night, nature took over. The babies decided that man was not their best friend, and they went off into the woods on their own. For two days Warren left food, but the man who was monitoring the hacking box said that adult raccoons were eating it, so Warren stopped the handouts.

We can only assume that the babies had finally returned to the wild. It was a long, hard row for them to hoe, but instinct does take over eventually. I see adult raccoons from time to time in my woods in the evenings and I wonder whether they were once the Wildlife Center babies. But I don't ask.

THE HOUSE THAT DISAPPEARED

In the spring, the eagles came back to the old nest for the twentieth year. Far, far back in the wilderness, the nest had served them well. This year the female added a stick here and there to reinforce it and repair any winter damage. The male brought sticks and food as the beginning of his courtship. Though they had been together at the same site for twenty years, they still went through the courtship rituals every year, the same as they had the year they had first built the nest.

It was atop an old snag in a small clearing. Years of use and repair had increased its size until it measured nearly ten feet across and could have held a man. Finally, satisfied with her labors, the female was ready. She flew up into the air with a shrill cry on strong wings and steadily rose in huge circles. The male followed. They rode the thermals, floating lazily, and then up they surged again, higher and higher until they were specks to a human eye. This was their mating flight which would end in copulation.

Once mated, the female laid her eggs and brooded, while the male hunted and brought food. In time, the eaglets pecked through their shells. There were three, a big family this year. Usually the eagles raised two young.

The man with the binoculars smiled as he saw the three small heads come up when the parents returned from fishing. They all seemed to be doing well. He was glad that the nest was active again this year. That meant the pair had wintered well and were still together. Pleased, Ron Eckstein, the Department of Natural Resources wildlife manager whose specialty was eagles, put the binoculars away, hoisted his backpack a bit more comfortably on his shoulders and started the long trek back to civilization. It had been a difficult trip, but it was worth it. All was well.

When the eaglets were about three weeks old, it began to rain. It wasn't a storm, just a gentle rain, but it went on all day and all night. The next day also started out as a dismal wet morning with more rain falling. The male eagle continued his hunting, but the female covered her young with sheltering wings. Periodically, she would stand up to shake the water from her great wings, and then would settle again over the young. Except for the warm dry circle her body protected, the nest was sodden. The weight of the water was added to the vast weight of the huge nest itself. The twenty-year-old underpinnings could no longer sustain the weight. One by one they cracked and gave way, adding to the pressure on the branches immediately around them. Others cracked and fell to the ground. The female bird was uneasy. Strange things were going on beneath her. She stood, looking around for danger, but could see none. More of the bottom of the nest gave way. Suddenly, the rest all collapsed at once and crashed to the ground. The female sprang into the air with a shriek. The male returned. Both sat on the bare snag. They seemed unable to comprehend what had happened. This is where their nest was. Here they would stay.

On the ground among the debris lay three eaglets. Two were unharmed, the third was dead. The two flopped around on the ground, emitting peeps that would ordinarily bring their parents promptly with food. None was forthcoming. Since birds are incapable of reasoning, they react to stimuli with inherent behavioral responses. When the nestlings peep for food, that is the stimulus to bring food to the nest. It is possible that the eagles were hunting after the nest disaster, but brought the food to where the nest had been. They were unable to make the mental jump that would have made them take the food to the young on the ground. The two youngsters went hungry.

A rabbit hunter, who had also watched the eagle nest for years, was the first to find the catastrophe. Fearful of engendering the wrath of the adults if he were to touch their offspring, and knowing that a full grown angry eagle was nothing to tamper with, the hunter elected instead to wait until he was near a phone to notify the Department of Natural Resources in Tomahawk. He then continued his hunting expedition.

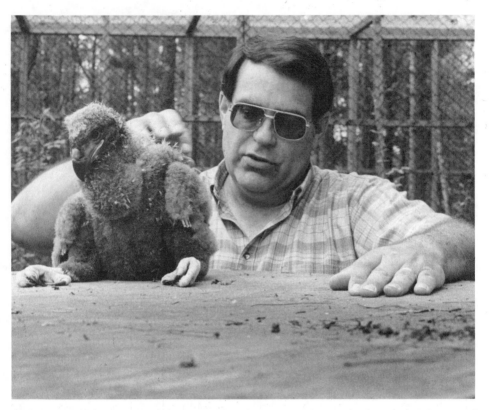

Warren feeds a baby eagle, standing behind it so the eaglet won't see him and imprint on humans.

THE HOUSE THAT DISAPPEARED

Chuck Sindalar of the DNR called the Wildlife Center. Would we take the babies until a "foster" nest could be found? Of course we would.

An eagle call to the Center sets everyone's heart beating a little faster. Naturally, the whole animal crew wanted to go, and naturally, we called Bob Baldwin, knowing that he would jump at the photo opportunity. He did. The Center crew was chosen. Dave went, of course, and two of the interns, and none of them had any idea of what they were getting into.

They met Chuck Sindalar at the Tomahawk ranger station and trucked into the woods on an old dirt trail. When they had been thoroughly bounced around, they stopped the truck for the simple reason that they had run out of road. It was now hiking time. They divided up the rescue boxes and gear and began a seemingly endless hike through the brush. What path there may have been was clogged with new spring growth. Their objective was not the nest site, but an old railroad spur left from the logging days. Transportation down that spur was by handcar which they took turns pumping. At last they reached the end of the spur, but still not the nest site.

"How did you ever find this nest when it was a nest?" one of the interns gasped.

"Fellow that hunts back here," replied Chuck. "He told us about it years ago. We've been monitoring it ever since. Lucky thing he was hunting yesterday. He found the mess."

The crew members again took up their burdens and walked behind Chuck, single file, deep into the woods. Finally at a small clearing, they located the nest site. The two adults were still in the area and shrieked and cackled warnings to the humans who were invading their territory.

The humans looked on the ground. There were the two eaglets, weak and dehydrated, but alive. Carefully, Dave put them in the carrying boxes as Bob Baldwin took pictures. For him, it was worth all the effort. For the Center, it would be worth it only if the babies could be saved.

The entire entourage, eaglets and all, started the long tortuous trip back.

Once at the Center, the eaglets were given emergency treatment. Fluids and food went down and they were put in a "nest" built by humans and placed next to Clawdia's cage so that they would constantly see an adult eagle and not lose sight of who they were. When they were fed, the person feeding stood behind them so that they would not associate humans and food and think a person was a parent.

Meanwhile, Ron Eckstein went out hunting for a foster nest to house them when they were strong enough to hold their own with foster siblings. He had been monitoring all the nests and knew where to look first. He found two suitable nests on the Rainbow Flowage. One nest contained a single eaglet and could easily take another of the same size. One of our babies went there and thrived. The second nest had two eaglets in it, but were of the right size to grow with ours. The second eaglet was placed in that nest.

And the adult eagles? What will happen to them? Next spring they will probably come back to the old snag and start a new nest in the same location. Maybe good for another twenty years?

THE BAT

The voice on the phone was young.

"Do you take bats?" It was a girl's voice.

"Yes, of course. Is it hurt?" I asked.

"It looks like it. It's just lying on the ground sort of fluttering. I think it's sick."

"Can you bring it in? Just use gloves and put it in a box. It won't hurt you."

"I can't. There's nobody home but me and it's a resort. I'm not supposed to leave in case someone comes in. Can you come? I don't want it to die."

The girl seemed genuinely concerned, which was a happy circumstance. Too many people when confronted with bats, sick or well, can think only of killing them.

"Of course I will come," I said. I knew this call was up to me. The whole back room gang was busy with baby feeding, and on top of that a new family of raccoon babies had been brought in and were being checked out. I picked up a nearly empty tissue box, a pair of gloves and told everyone I would be back with a sick bat shortly.

"Bat!" screamed one of the interns. I sighed. It was the predictable response.

"Yes, bat!" I repeated and left.

As I drove through Minocqua, I had to stop while every piece of fire equipment screamed out of the side street and headed down highway 51. I was right behind them, fully aware that fire truck chasing was a no-no, but after all that is where I was going, too.

WILDLIFE HOSPITAL

The resort was in Hazelhurst, a few miles down the road. As we neared my turnoff, I thought the fire trucks would continue down the highway. They did not. They turned down my road right ahead of me, and there was nothing to do but follow. There were several forks in the road we were on. I was to keep bearing right. At any time, the fire trucks could have gone left, but they did not. We screamed down the roads together. By now the firemen on the truck were glancing back to see who was following them. It was not until I actually turned down the driveway to the resort that I left the parade. Never did a patient have such an escort for its ambulance.

The girl was waiting for me in the big yard under the huge pine trees

"There he is." She pointed to a small black lump on the ground.

I put on one glove and hunkered down to get a better look. The little creature was quivering all over. Suddenly, my nose told me what his trouble was.

"Have you been spraying for bugs?"

"Yes, the men came this morning."

"He's been poisoned by the spray. His little lungs can't take it. I'll take him out of here and into better air, but I can't make any promises. We'll do what we can."

The girl was near tears. "We did it to him, didn't we?"

"You didn't know. Don't feel bad. But next year depend on your bat friends and all their relatives to take care of your bug population. They can eat more mosquitoes than you can kill with a spray, AND they do it all summer long!"

"I'll tell my dad. Somehow I don't mind killing mosquitoes, but I don't like killing animals."

I was busy picking the little bat up and putting him in the tissue box. I wanted to get him out of the sprayed area.

As we walked to the car, I gave her something else to tell her father.

"You see, when you spray, it kills everything. Good bugs and nuisances. Damsel flies and dragon flies eat insects, too. The praying mantis also eats other insects. Then the birds and mice and small owls who also eat insects may eat the poisoned ones and get sick like your little bat here. It's really best just to leave nature alone. It sort of takes care of itself."

I got in the car. "Thanks for calling me. We'll do the best we can for the little fellow."

I drove off, leaving her where I found her, standing in the yard under the big pines.

As I approached the road, a big orange Department of Natural Resources flatbed truck roared by with a bulldozer on its back. Obviously, the fire was a wildfire and meant trouble. The woods were dry. I drove back to the Center thinking about all the wildlife that would be affected by the fire. A whole small ecological unit would be destroyed and would not be re-established for years thereafter. But in a way, the spraying at the resort had done the same thing on a smaller scale. It would be a long time before the area was safe for insects, mammals, and birds. Nature rebuilds, but slowly, with the seasons. Man can destroy in a day.

When I got back to the Center, the back room had calmed down a bit, and Dave looked over my little patient.

"Probably an oil spray," he said. "If it's in his lungs, it will just have to absorb and dissipate. He'll be all right if we can just keep him alive that long. I'll put him in one of those bird cages and keep him outside."

One of the interns brought him a cage. Gently, Dave placed the small bat and his tissue bed on the floor of the cage.

WILDLIFE HOSPITAL

"We'll need some meal worms in here for him to eat."

The intern headed for the mealworm aquarium, and had just removed the top when Dave said, "Oh, oh. Never mind. He died."

I felt a lump in my throat and left the room as Dave reached for the small, still body.

THE RAT RUN

The back room or treatment room at the Center bears a strong resemblance to a kitchen. On one wall is a bank of cabinets, below which is a regular kitchen counter, and at one end of the counter is a sink. We wash dishes just like you do.

Across from the sink is a refrigerator, just as it would be in any kitchen, but there the resemblance stops. What you keep in your refrigerator and what we keep in ours differ mightily! The freezer contains some frozen fish and some wrapped venison — possibly no difference there. But also in our freezer are packages of rats and mice. Everyday, the volunteer who works in the back room removes sufficient rats, mice, fish and venison from the freezer for the next day's feeding before he or she leaves. This goes into the refrigerator to be thawed overnight and be ready for dinner the following day. Woe be unto the volunteer who forgets! Dinner then has to be thawed in the microwave, and I am sure you can all imagine how that odor permeates the Center!

The volunteer feeding the animals must sometimes cut food up to get the right number of ounces for a particular patient. We lose some volunteers that way since not everyone is up to cutting rats in half! People who would not quiver at splitting a chicken go all to pieces when they are faced with splitting a rat.

The mice and rats are donated by a genetics laboratory. When the researchers have finished with a project, they call us and let us know that a certain number of rats and/or mice will be available and will we please pick them up. Since we are deeply grateful for their contribution to our animals, it behooves us to accommodate them as quickly as possible.

One day a mouse call came to the Center.

"The lab just called. Who can make a mouse run?" I asked of anyone within earshot. Since the Center is so small, everyone could hear me easily. It developed that Dave could not go as there

115

was no volunteer coming in the next day and he would have to clean and feed. Tony had a program in Merrill. That meant that either Bill or I was elected. Since Bill was the Director, it seemed better if he stayed and minded the store while I went after the mice. Besides, I had a late Christmas present for my grandchildren and I could deliver that at the same time. I volunteered.

I called the lab back.

"This is Sybil. I'll be picking up the mice and will be there about noon tomorrow."

"It's rats, this time. Will that be a problem?"

"Not at all," I said in my abysmal ignorance. "I'll bring some coolers."

"Will you be driving the truck?" Sharon asked.

"No, my station wagon. There should be plenty of room."

"Ok, we'll see you tomorrow around noon." We both hung up.

Before I went home that afternoon, I took the two coolers out of the storage room and put them in my car with a pile of newspapers. I had been on a mouse run before and had put the neat little packages of frozen mice side by side in the coolers until they were full. The remaining packages I put between the coolers wrapped in newspapers for insulation. I was now prepared.

I planned to leave early in the morning.

That night I called my son and invited myself for brunch the following day. Since he is a writer and editor who works at home, he could adjust his schedule to fit in a brief visit. If Jeannie, his wife, could get away from the office, I might even get to see her, too. The girls would be home, since Christmas vacation was not yet over. It was going to be a great mouse run!

I left before seven in the morning. Northern Wisconsin mornings in the dead of winter are not exactly warm, and it was a while before the heater generated enough heat to make driving comfortable. The rest of the ride was uneventful and I arrived at John's house shortly before eleven. The girls finally had their last Christmas present and we sat down to a cozy brunch. Jeannie came in and joined us halfway through and it was a thoroughly successful visit.

Then it was noon and time for me to pick up my cargo. The lab was not far from the house and was an easy drive. I stopped at the front office and went in.

"Hello! I'm Sybil from the Wildlife Center about the mice."

"Oh, yes. We've added more rats to the load. It's really rats this time, you know," said Sharon.

"Yes, I understand." I said, not really understanding at all!

"You will have to pick them up from the dock. That is around behind this building and past the lab to the left. You can't miss it."

"OK, fine. Thank you very much." I left the office and climbed back into the car, still in blissful ignorance.

I found the loading dock without any trouble. It was easily identifiable since a load of fifty pound sacks of sunflower seeds had just been delivered.

"Wow!" I thought. "Their animals must eat a lot!"

A man came through the door. I identified myself.

"You got a truck?" he inquired.

"No, I just brought my wagon." He looked at me and I looked at him. He seemed to feel that something was wrong. I couldn't fathom what it could be.

"Well, let's load it then."

"Right," I said. Then I watched in horror as he picked up one of the huge bags of what I had thought were seeds. I counted the bags. Sixteen.

"How many rats are in those bags?" I asked weakly.

"One hundred, give or take a few," he answered as he put another bag into the back cargo area of the wagon. He was standing them up three abreast. Each kraft bag had an inner plastic bag of rats, tied securely. Four rows fitted neatly into the back.

"How much does a rat weigh?" I asked weakly.

"Oh, maybe pound and a half average. Some big ones two pounds or more." He peered into the back seat. "OK I put a coupla bags in here?"

"What? Oh yes. Fine."

Three more bags went into the back seat.

"There's still one bag. Front seat?"

I thought about two hundred miles with a front seat companion that was a bag of rats. I thought about what would happen if I were in an accident and any of the bags burst. I thought about being stopped for a traffic violation and having the State Patrol ask me what was in the bags. I swallowed bravely and said, "Fine!"

The last bag was loaded and the man said, "Car's riding pretty low."

I looked at the mudguards. They were touching the ground with some to spare.

"You'd better drive slow. Don't go over any bumps. Should have brought a truck." The man waved and returned to the building.

There was nothing to do but go home. I got into the car and started back. I did drive slowly, and I was careful about bumps. It was about one-thirty when I left. Under more favorable circumstances I would have been home by five. As it was, at five I was still on the road just north of Merrill and it was getting dark. I still had an hour's driving ahead of me. Time to turn on the lights. I did, but they did not! The little red light came on on the dashboard to inform me that the headlights had suddenly given up the ghost. Impossible! I turned them off and turned them on again. Still the little red light. I didn't believe it and pulled over to the side of the road to see for myself. The red light was right! I had no headlights!

Luckily, the parking lights still worked. I started up again and drove faster, never mind the load. I had to get home. I found a car with headlights and cuddled up close behind it. The driver must have thought I was an atrocious driver but I needed the protection of headlights for oncoming cars. His would have to serve. They did serve until the Harshaw turn off. He turned off, no doubt relieved that I did not follow. But I was bereft! The night was darker than ever and I still had miles to go. There was nothing to do but drive.

By the time I reached my own turn-off I was clutching the wheel tightly and felt as if my eyes were sticking out of my head from trying to see the road. Oncoming cars beeped their horns at me and flashed their lights. I would have given anything to be able to turn mine on for them, but I was helpless.

There was no question of my driving through town with no lights. I headed for home and called Bill.

"Hi! I'm home and I have the rats, but my lights are off and will you pick them up?"

It took Bill a while to decipher my code, but he finally did and said he would be right down with the truck. I was never so glad to see anyone. He was my knight in shining armor when he drove up in the Center truck. We parked back to back and he transferred sixteen 150 lb. bags into the truck and drove away...slowly, watching for bumps.

I parked my wagon in the garage and apologized to it before closing the door and giving it a long night's rest. I, however, had a hard time getting to sleep that night.

And that is a rat run!

THE STORY OF MARLIE

The call came in routinely. There was nothing at all in the call to warn of the little drama that was to follow.

"Do you take care of birds?" the woman asked.

"Wild birds," I answered thinking she might have a canary, a parakeet, a cockatiel or some other exotic.

"Oh, it's wild," she assured me. "I think it's a little hawk."

"That sounds like our kind of bird," I laughed. "What's wrong?"

"It's been chewing on its wing. It hurt the wing about a week ago, and it keeps pecking on the sore place. I think it's getting infected. What should I put on it?" she asked.

"Where are you? Would you like to bring it in, or do you want us to pick it up?"

"Oh, no! I just want to know what to put on it. I'm going to keep the bird," she answered.

"I'm sorry, but if you have a hawk, that is a bird of prey, and you are not allowed to keep it unless you have a permit. May I have your name please?" I asked the routine question.

"Certainly not!" she exploded, and hung up.

I was left with my mouth open holding a silent phone. I shrugged and hung up.

"What was that?" asked Dave, who was sorting through slides at the table.

"Some woman with a little hawk. It has a bad wing, but she wants to keep it. She hung up on me," I explained.

"Probably a kestrel," said Dave, and went back to his sorting.

Several days later, the same voice called. This time I said, "Let me give you to our rehabilitator. He can advise you better than I," and I called Dave.

A short while later, he walked out of the back room looking chastened. "She hung up on me, too," he admitted. "But the poor bird sounds like it's in bad shape. She was really teed off when I told her we didn't examine birds over the phone. She sure doesn't want to bring it in." He shrugged and went back to the rehab area.

The third call was mine, and I got the brunt of the woman's anger.

"You're a wildlife hospital, aren't you? You take care of hurt birds, don't you? My bird is getting worse and worse and you won't even tell me what to do for it. It wouldn't hurt YOU to help it out!"

"Please," I pleaded, "For the sake of the bird, please bring it in, or let us come and get it."

"Could I have it back?" she demanded.

"Only if you have a permit to keep a bird of prey. We'd lose our license if we let you keep it illegally."

Wham! went the phone. I hung up.

I walked into the back room. "That must be one sick kestrel, to have her calling like that," I said to Dave. "What would happen if you just told her to put something or other on it? It's the bird that's getting the short end of the stick."

"How would you like a doctor to prescribe to you over the phone?

Think!" said Dave.

"You're right," I admitted, "But I feel sorry for the bird."

The following Sunday close to four o'clock when we close, a car swooped into the parking lot and made a half circle in front of the door. I walked around the desk to greet whoever was coming in in such a rush, when the car door opened and a woman put a box on the ground in front of our door. In a half-second she slammed her door, and the car took off in a spray of gravel. I was not smart enough to look for a license number.

"Dave!" I called.

Dave came up to the front.

"What's up?" he asked.

"I think we have a new patient. That box was just left here, but the people took off."

Dave went out and retrieved the box. He set it on the table and we both looked inside. Dave reached in and gently pulled out a small hawk. It wasn't a kestrel. I had never seen one like it. Dave, meanwhile, started cussing under his breath as he saw the badly infected wing. The odor was horrendous.

"A merlin!" he breathed. "A merlin! And she wouldn't bring it in!" "There's no saving that wing. She'll never fly again." He carried the little merlin to the back room to do what he could for her until the vets came in in the morning and the wing could be amputated. Bill was out of his office by now, and he carried the box into the back room for disposal.

"We'll have to call the DNR in the morning," Dave said. "They'll want to know about this. If there were only some way to find out where the woman found the bird. They don't nest in Wisconsin. If she really did find a nest that this young one fell from, that's a real breakthrough." Bill was taking the papers out of the box.

"Oh, oh," he said. "Pay dirt! Look here!" He held up one of the newspapers. "She gets her newspapers through the mail. Guess what's on this one!"

Dave grinned his wide grin. "It wouldn't be a name and address, now, would it?"

"Bingo!" said Bill.

The Department of Natural Resources notified the woman that they would not prefer charges for keeping a bird of prey illegally, if she would tell them where she got the bird. It was a fair exchange, both from the point of view of the DNR and the woman concerned. We were not notified of the outcome. The only loser was the little merlin.

As Dave suspected, Marty Smith said the wing would have to come off. After a long series of antibiotics, Marlie, the merlin, healed and became one of our education birds. She had her cage on the trail, and her story was told over and over to emphasize the need for prompt treatment of injuries, and the fine points of the law concerning birds of prey. Although she was not a free bird in the wild population, she helped educate the public on merlins, and the work of the Center. Still, it would have been better if she had been brought in at the first telephone call. Maybe the wing could have healed. Maybe she could have returned to the wild. Maybe there would be merlins nesting in Wisconsin.

The Wildlife Center has other birds like Marlie which are unable to be released, and which serve as education birds. Education is an important function of the Center, and thousands of people have learned about wildlife from touring our facility, especially the Judi Lowmiller Trail. Please join me as I take a family on a tour in the next section of the book. As the family stops to look at the various permanent residents, I'll take some time to tell you their stories.

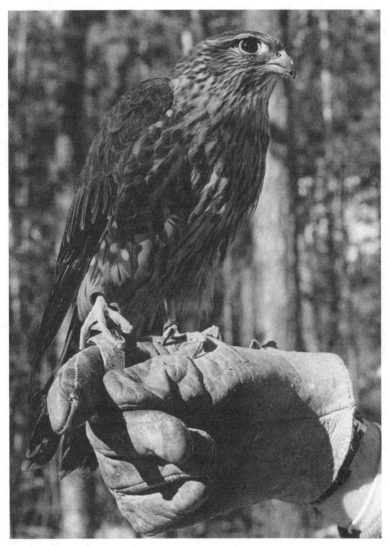

Marlie the Merlin shows us her "good side."

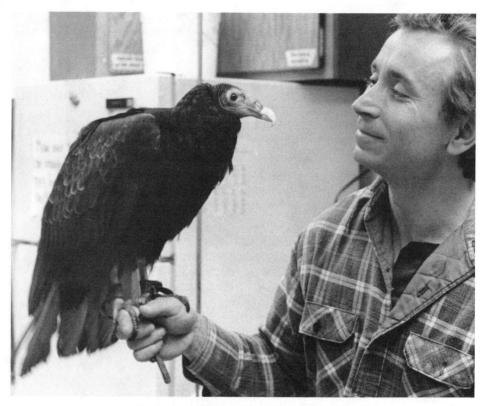

Dave shares a private joke with Hortense, the turkey vulture.

PART II:
THE PERMANENT
RESIDENTS:
OUR "EDUCATION"
ANIMALS

A TOUR OF
THE CENTER

"Hello. May I help you?"

It was a family this time, a mother, father and three children, ranging in age from about a six year old boy, through a slightly older girl and topped by another boy about twelve.

"Can we look around?" the mother asked.

"Certainly, I'll give you the 'grand tour'. Will you sign the guest book, please?" I waited while each member of the family signed.

"Can we see the animals?" the small boy asked.

"Some of them," I answered. "Remember that we are a hospital and a hospital doesn't show its patients."

"Why not?" he persisted. "I want to see the animals."

"It's a hospital for WILD animals. We have to keep them wild so that they can go back and live in the wild. We can't let them get used to people. And anyway, being around people bothers them. They get frightened. Then they don't get well as fast as they should." I could see that I was fighting a losing battle. "I can show you some of our education animals. They are used to people and it doesn't bother them."

The boy fell silent, appeased. By now the whole family was ready for the tour.

"Will you come this way, please." I led them down the hallway between our building and the Foster Smith Animal Hospital. The two buildings, the hall and a solid board fence enclose a courtyard where, in summer, we keep orphaned and injured fawns. There were two out there at this time, and as luck would have it, a volunteer was bottle-feeding them. Linda had a bottle in each hand, and both fawns were busy, tails flapping happily, legs braced.

"Awww! Look at them! Aren't they darling?" The family was enthralled. They were standing at the big, one-way window that allowed them to look out, but did not allow the fawns to see them.

"These are patients," I told the small boy, "but they can't see us through this special window. So that makes it all right to look at them. The one on the right was orphaned. He was found near a doe that had been killed by a car. The other one was hit by a car, herself. See the white cast around her front leg?" The boy nodded. "That leg was broken and Dr. Smith put a steel pin in the bone to hold it straight so it will heal properly. When it is well, the steel pin will be removed and the fawn can be released. Of course, we have to take care of her until she can take care of herself. She's just a baby now. We'll let them both go in the fall."

"Won't they get shot?" asked mother anxiously.

"Not where we release them," I smiled. "We take them up to Dairyman's Country Club near Boulder Junction, north of here. They have ten thousand acres, seven lakes, and no hunting. The deer herd comes in for dinner every night. The Marquardts feed them at the lodge."

"Sounds like the right place for them," said the father.

"Can I feed them?" asked the little girl, longingly.

"No, I'm sorry. Only our animal volunteers feed them. Watch Linda. She isn't talking to them, or petting them. She is just holding the bottles. When they have finished, she will leave. We are very careful not to make pets out of the animals, even though it is very hard with some of the babies. We are around them only to feed and clean them. It's good that we have two fawns. They keep each other company, and since deer are herd animals, they need each other."

WILDLIFE HOSPITAL

"Who pays for all this?" asked the father.

"People do," I replied. "We are a nonprofit corporation supported entirely by memberships and donations — no state or federal funds—just caring people. Sometimes for special projects we get money from a foundation, but the daily operation of the Center depends on people."

"Excuse us, please." Dave and Jacquie were coming through the hall to the animal hospital. In Dave's arms was a great horned owl which had been brought in yesterday and was now ready to have his broken wing set. They disappeared through the door.

"What happened to that bird?" asked the older boy.

"We don't know. It was found by the side of the road, and so we are guessing it was a car-strike."

"What was it?" he asked.

"That was a great horned owl. They are very common around here." By now the aura of skunk permeated the air. Strange expressions came over all five visitor faces.

"Yuuck!" said the small boy. "It stinks!"

"That's the owl. They have a very poor sense of smell, and the skunk smell doesn't bother them. They eat it for dinner. Nearly every great horned owl that is brought in smells of skunk. We look them over and keep them in OUTSIDE cages! Guess why? Now, if you will please go past the reception desk and turn down the middle hallway, there's another window."

The family obediently followed directions and stopped in front of the one-way window into the flight room.

"This is the room where we keep birds who are learning to fly, or need to exercise their wings after recovering from an injury."

"What's in there?" the girl asked. "They are all fuzzy."

"Those are baby barred owls. Three of them are from one nest and two from another. Loggers brought them in after they had cut the nest trees down."

"Couldn't they just leave those trees alone?" asked the girl.

"They didn't know the nests were there until after the trees were cut. Then they felt bad and brought the babies in here."

"What do they eat? Skunks, too?"

"These are just babies. They eat mice."

"Where do you get enough mice to feed five owls?" the mother wanted to know.

"A laboratory raises them for research and when the research is complete, the mice are humanely killed, frozen and we get them free as a donation. Every day the animal volunteer takes enough mice out of the freezer for the next day. Many of our animals eat mice. Rats, too."

"Yuuck!" said the little boy.

"It isn't 'Yuuck' if you are an owl," I said. "For them it is 'Yummy'."

Linda, who by now had finished with the fawns, brought in a tray of mice for the five baby owls. The family watched, fascinated.

"You came at a good time," I said. "Feeding time. You can watch them eat."

"How can they eat those mice?" asked the mother. "Don't you cut them into small pieces?"

"Watch," I answered.

One baby approached the mouse laid out on the perch closest to him. He hunched his stubby wings over it and placed a possessive foot on it. Glaring at his roommates, he grabbed the mouse's head in his beak and raised it skyward. One gulp and the head disappeared. Another gulp and the chest vanished, a third gulp, and nothing was left but the tail hanging out of the side of his beak. One more gulp and that was gone.

"He ate it whole!" breathed the older boy.

"Yuuck!" said the little one.

The family watched a second, then a third mouse disappeared as the baby owls ate their dinners. I then suggested we move over to the south window from which we could see Teton, our golden eagle.

"Teton is not a native of Wisconsin. He comes from Wyoming."

"How old is he?" asked the father. "Is that his adult plumage?"

"Yes, he is an adult. But we don't know how old he is. He was an adult when we got him."

"How did you get him all the way from Wyoming?" asked the mother.

"They didn't have a rehabilitation center in Wyoming where he could be kept. They heard about us through one of our former interns who was skiing out there and that is how we got him."

TETON'S STORY

Hank dialed the phone. "Say, Ed, you got any gas in that airplane of yours?"

"Oh, Hi, Hank. Sure. She's gassed up and ready to go. What's on your mind?"

"There's a couple of eagles flying over my spread the past coupla days. I got lambs coming, and I don't feel real friendly toward those birds."

"Gotcha!" said Ed. "You come on over and we'll take care of them."

"Thanks. I'll bring Herb Mosely. He's a good shot."

"Right. See you." Ed hung up the phone.

The pair of golden eagles soared over the plains of Wyoming. They were young, newly mated. They would stay together for life. The male had staked out this territory and had brought his mate here for nesting. They had found a suitable spot in a nearby canyon, and were riding the thermals as they searched for prey. Their favorite food was the cottontail rabbit, plentiful on the grassy plains. Soon they would gather the sticks with which they would construct their nest — a marvelous feat of engineering which would be the nucleus of many nests to come as they added to and rebuilt it each year. The nest would someday extend twenty feet across and weigh several hundred pounds. Now, it was simply a site on top of an outcropping which pleased them both.

The female spotted a rabbit and suddenly dived to the ground. As she flew close to the earth, her powerful talons grasped the rabbit and lifted it as the talons squeezed tightly to suffocate the prey. She landed near the nest site and the male joined her. She shared her prey, only because he was her mate and they were

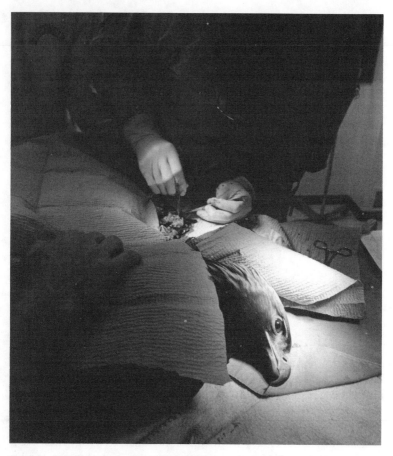

Teton, a golden eagle, was shot by a rancher in Wyoming, requiring surgery to repair her wing.

still courting. A strange eagle would have had short shrift. First they ate the contents of the rabbit's stomach and intestines. Thus, they got their veggies as the rabbits were vegetarians. In the same way the lion, tiger, and other predators obtain the vitamins and minerals they need, even though they are meat eaters. The eagles then tore apart the rest of their prey while holding it in their powerful talons.

Once finished, they again took to the air. One cottontail was not enough for two hungry eagles.

After a time, the male dived down to the ground and captured a big jack rabbit. He did not have the quick recovery that the female had had. The jackrabbit outweighed the two- and-a-half-pound cottontail by an equal amount, and the male eagle, strong as he was, had a difficult time getting off the ground with his huge prey. The female descended and the two eagles again shared the prey, this time on the ground. Thoroughly sated, the birds rose into the air again, flying more slowly since they were both heavy with food. It sometimes happened that they ate so well that they were unable to fly and would have to wait until the food digested, sometimes for several hours. They were now no longer hunting. They flew playfully, just enjoying each other's company.

They were interrupted in their flight by the approach of a small airplane. They gave up their play and headed away from the plane and down into the canyon. The airplane followed. The birds flew higher. The plane followed. The birds slipped to the left and turned. The plane banked and turned after them. The plane had no trouble keeping up with the heavy birds. Once the plane was alongside the eagles, two puffs of smoke came from the opened window. The female eagle fell like a stone. The male turned over and over as he tried to recover flight with a severely damaged wing. The airplane turned and went back along the canyon and disappeared. The male landed on the canyon floor and flopped helplessly, until exhaustion overcame him and he lay still.

Then out of the sky a second plane appeared, with the blue and

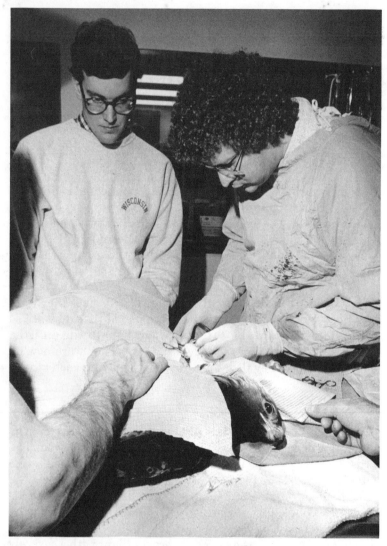

Tony looks on as Marty prepares to amputate part of Teton's wing.

white insignia of the U.S. Fish and Game Service and "Patrol" written on the underside of each wing. It streaked down the canyon, following the first plane, and also disappeared.

Several hours later, a man climbed down the canyon with a pack on his back. When he got to the canyon floor, he began criss-crossing from one side to the other, searching. There was no movement. He looked up and took his bearings again. Then he spoke into a walkie talkie unit. "I don't see it anywhere. I think I am right. Fly over and give me a wag when you get to where you saw them go down."

The plane with the blue and white insignia soon circled over-head. Then a wing dipped, and the plane flew on. The man on the ground changed direction and again criss-crossed the canyon. Suddenly, there was movement to his right. The man stood still and waited. Again a slight movement. The man moved slowly. It could be the eagle, or it could be a mountain lion. He was taking no chances until his eyes could identify the animal. After his long rest, the wounded eagle again tried to fly. His struggles confirmed his identity.

"I found him! Looks like he was shot in the wing. He can't fly. I'll bring him up."

The man approached the frantic bird and threw a blanket over him. Then, taking gloves from his pack, he carefully wrapped the blanket around the bird, being sure to fold the wings neatly to keep damage to a minimum. The eagle clutched the blanket with his talons, enabling the man to put him in a stout animal carry-all with a drawstring top. He fastened the bag to his backpack with the buckles on the sides, and he was ready to start the long climb up the canyon.

"Bad shape," said the vet. "A lot of pellets in there. Right on the joint, too. I don't know." He put the radiograph down and shook his head. "They may have to take that part of the wing off. He'll never fly again."

The wounded eagle and the capture of his human predators was

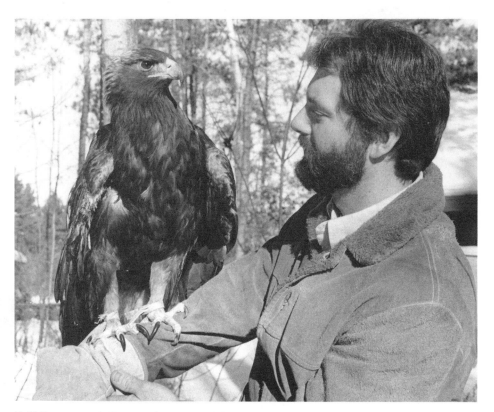

Bill Bauer with Teton, the new golden eagle from Wyoming

news. Among those who read with outrage the story of the wanton hunting of a protected species was a former intern at the Northwoods Wildlife Center. He had come out west to ski in the mountains. He interrupted his sport long enough to make several phone calls. One call went to the Wildlife Center to explain about the eagle. Another went to the U.S. Fish and Wildlife Service to explain about the Wildlife Center. The wheels were set in motion and the eagle made one more flight. This time he was aboard a Frontier Airlines plane which flew him without charge to Milwaukee, where he was met by Bill and Dave from the Wildlife Center. He next traveled in the Center truck to northern Wisconsin, which would be his home from then on. The Wyoming vet had been right. The wing could not be saved. Marty performed the amputation. Teton, the disabled golden eagle is now a permanent resident at the Center, on loan from the state of Wyoming.

The canyon lies quiet. There is no nest on the outcropping. No eaglets learn to fly on the thermals that rise above the canyon. The cottontail and jack rabbits eat the grass that could be feeding the rancher's sheep. The turkey vulture which fed on the eagle carcass was the only winner in this tragedy, and nature is again diminished by man.

I continued the tour as the family watched the golden eagle through the window.

"We started out feeding Teton rats and mice like the owls, but one day we ran out, and we looked in the freezer for something he could eat. We found some venison that a woman had given us when she cleaned out her freezer. When Teton tasted that he decided it was the best thing he ever had and since then he has refused to eat anything else!"

"How do you get it? Does everybody clean out freezers for him?" the mother laughed.

"No. We call the DNR when we get low, and ask them for the next road killed deer that is reported. Then when they call, we have to hurry before someone else gets there first. Mostly, we win, but

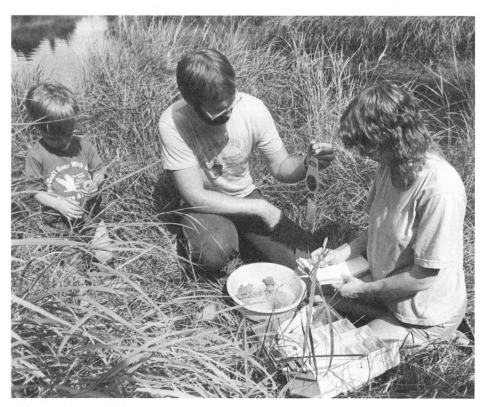

Kevin and Cass Brewster weigh young wood turtles, with help from a small volunteer.

sometimes when we get there, the deer is gone. When we do get them, Dave is usually the one stuck with the job of butchering it and putting the pieces down in the freezer. All that work for one spoiled eagle!"

"The pond area which you see out the window beyond Teton is where we kept the wood turtle project. The Rice Foundation funded that and Kevin Brewster was the herpetologist who did all the work." I turned to the smaller boy. "Can you guess where the turtles spent the winters?"

"I don't know," he shrugged.

"They hibernate, don't they?" asked the father.

"Yes, but at the Wildlife Center, we couldn't just leave these rare turtles outside. We brought them in and kept them in the refrigerator!"

"In the refrigerator!"

"Yes. Each turtle had his or her own tub with a little water in it. There were seven and the tubs just fitted fine on the shelves. Every week, Kevin and his wife, Cass, would come in and weigh them to be sure they were all right. Then they would change their water and they would be all set for another week."

"That's weird!" said the girl.

"Where are they now?" asked the smaller boy. "I don't see any."

"They have all been released," I explained. "The research has been completed and Kevin is writing it up for the Herpetological Society. While he was still observing them, he let them go with radio telemetry units attached to their shells so that he could follow them and see what they did. He was trying to find out why they were endangered, and why there were not lots of wood turtles around."

"Did he find out?" asked the girl.

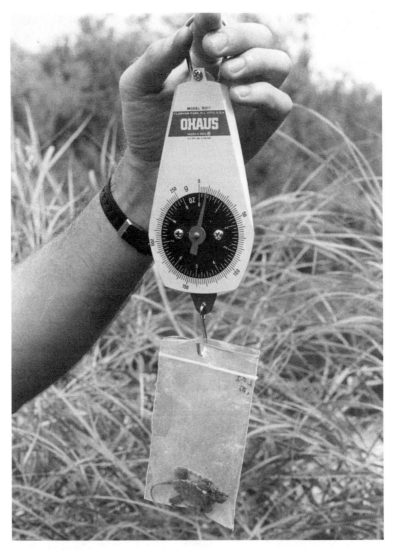

A crude but effective method is employed to weigh baby wood turtles.

"We won't know until he gets all his material together and writes it up. Then we'll know all about the wood turtles." I turned toward the door. "Would you like to go out on the trail and see the other animals?"

"Can we pet them?" asked the girl longingly.

"Sorry, no." I knew just how she felt. Part of getting to know anything is touching it. You want to feel its texture, its weight, its surface. It's hard not to touch. "Let's go out on the trail now. Wait. I have to get a key."

"Do you always keep it locked, or are we the first ones?" asked the father.

"Both, today. Yes, we always keep it locked, and yes, you are our first visitors of the day. We keep it locked because we are not licensed as a zoo, where people can browse through the place by themselves." I explained as we walked through the door and out onto the parking lot toward the Judi Lowmiller Trail. "We are a rehabilitation facility, and if we show you some of our animals, we must always escort you and tell you about what you are seeing. It's supposed to be an educational tour. I hope it turns out that way for you!"

"We've learned a lot already," said the mother smiling. "You must be doing your job."

I smiled back. "Thanks. Here we are."

The padlock, as usual, was hard for me to open. I wrestled with it a moment before it decided to separate. I opened the big double gate and went through first.

"I'll lead, if you please, and then I can talk to you better about the animals you are looking at. Please close the gate when everyone is in." I stopped between the sides of the trail where there was nothing to see, and turned to them.

"All the animals you will see on the trail are disabled in some

143

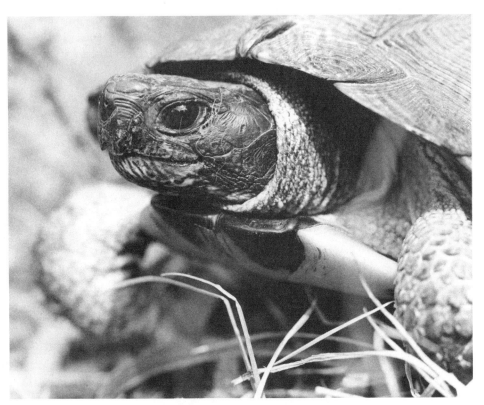

A fully grown wood turtle is a cooperative, if wary subject for Bob's camera.

way. Some have been physically injured and haven't healed properly so that they cannot be released into the wild and be able to take care of themselves. Others were psychologically damaged by being imprinted with man when they were babies, and they no longer identify with their own species. In most cases this imprinting is irreversible and the birds cannot survive in the wild."

I turned to go on, but the oldest boy had a question. "How do they get imprinted in the first place?"

"Usually, by being raised by a human. When a baby bird first opens its eyes and looks around, it knows who it is by seeing who is feeding it. Mostly, a baby eagle would see the eagle parents, or a baby hawk would see hawks, but when a person raises a baby bird, that is what the baby sees, and the little bird figures he's 'people'." I paused. "Or that people are birds. And after that, he just never changes his mind."

"Do you have some that are imprinted?"

"Yes. I'll tell you about them when we get there." I moved on. "Now this first cage is our song bird cage. See the fine mesh? We made it that way so that even the tiniest birds couldn't get out. But do you know what happened?"

"What?" said the smaller boy.

"One day we had an injured purple finch. It had run into a window. Nothing was broken, and so we put him out here to recover for a while. The next day, when we came to feed him, the purple finch was there, and a chickadee was with him! Neither one could get out, but it was certain that the little chickadee had gotten in! And the NEXT day when we brought the seeds out, can you guess what had happened?"

"What?" asked the boy.

"There was a purple finch, a chickadee, and a junco! It was just like The House That Jack Built. Something new was added every

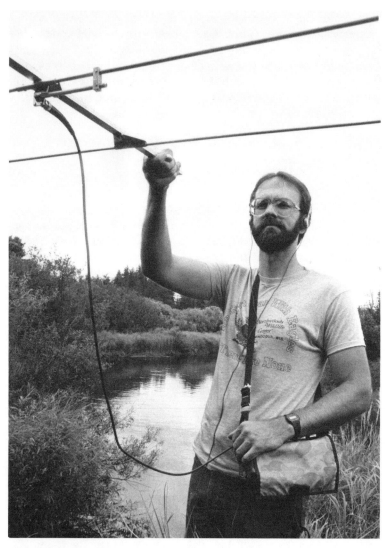

Kevin Brewster looks for his "traveling" wood turtles with radio telemetry gear.

day. The finch was fine by then, and so we just opened the door and let everybody go. We still haven't found how they got in and we looked over the whole cage. The only possibility is that tiny knot hole in the board part of the cage."

I moved down the trail a bit. "Now, if you look through the window on the other side, you will see into the pond area. See, right by the tree near the flowering bush on the other side......."

"I see it! It's a great blue heron! We have one on our lake!" The girl was all excited. "What's wrong with him?"

"He is actually a patient, but he can't see you through the dark glass. Just like inside. He swallowed a fishhook that someone left out with a minnow on it. It showed very clearly on the X-ray. Dr. Smith operated and removed it, and the heron is doing just fine. He has been released several times."

"What do you mean? Are there complications?"

"No not at all. You see that there is no mesh over the top of this enclosure. Whenever he feels ready to leave, he is free to go. But he is a little spoiled."

"How do you mean?" asked the mother.

"We have been dumping minnows into that blue wading pool for him to eat, and it's easy pickin's for him when he is hungry. He flies away, but if he doesn't do very well fishing on his own, he comes back for a handout. He's a moocher!"

After everyone had seen our semi-resident heron, we all moved down the trail.

"This is Sugar. She is an American kestrel. She is the smallest of the hawks. They used to call them sparrow hawks but that was a kind of derogatory name, so they changed it to kestrel. Actually, kestrel is the proper name, but no one ever called them that. She is one of the falcons. You see, there are three kinds of hawks and they are easy to remember if you think of FAB laundry

147

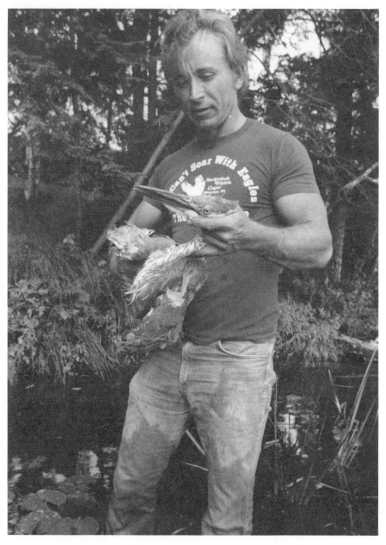

Dave rescues a Great Blue Heron that has swallowed a fishhook.

detergent. F is for falcon, which has pointed wings and is very quick and maneuverable. The kestrel is one, and the merlin, which is slightly larger, is another, and you have all heard of the peregrine falcon which they are attempting to establish in the big cities to control the pigeon population. Falcons eat other birds for dinner. The peregrine was even called the 'duck hawk' at one time. So you can remember F is for falcons. The A is for accipiters. The goshawk is one of those. Their wings are stubby, and they are a little heavier bird, and not so quick as the falcons. The B is for buteo, like the broadwing hawk and the red-tailed hawk. Their wings are longer, and also stubby, and they tend to prey more on mammals rather than birds....

There you have all of them: falcon, accipiter, and buteo — FAB. Can you remember that?"

"No!" said the smaller boy honestly. The others just smiled.

"They have some peregrine falcons in Minneapolis," the father said.

"Yes, and also in Chicago, Detroit, Milwaukee, New York, and many other cities. They want them to become accustomed to nesting on skyscrapers. Actually, they are cliff-nesters, so that tall buildings would be a 'natural'. There is just one thing the planners overlooked the first year!"

"What was that?" asked the father.

"They did not realize that the peregrines choose a protected spot on the cliff, so that the nest is safe from predators. In the open on a flat roof, they are an open invitation to any animal who is hungry. The peregrine nests have been a bonanza for great horned owls feeding their own babies. The young peregrines were delicious!"

"Can't they do anything to stop that?"

"They did, of course, when they realized what was happening. They built sheltered areas for the peregrines to nest in. Things

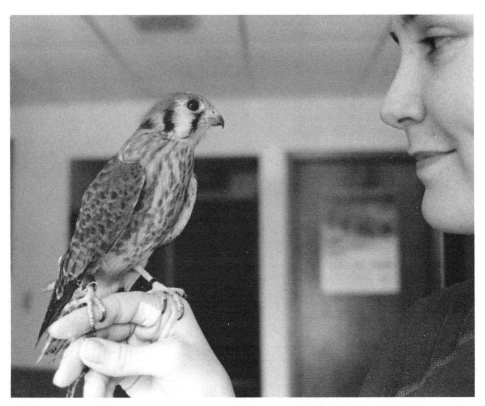

Jacquie DeBauche holds Sugar, the American kestrel, on her finger.

are looking up. The owls will have a harder time from now on."

"Live and learn," commented the mother.

"This little kestrel also eats birds for dinner. She flies above the bird she wants to catch and is quick enough to outfly and outmaneuver anything she goes after. When she is ready to make her strike, she dive bombs her prey. She closes her wings and just drops. It is called going into a stoop. Kestrels have been clocked at fifty to sixty miles per hour in the stoop. When she gets right above her prey, she spreads her wings to put on the brakes and puts out her talons. ZAP! She has it, and the feathers fly. The kestrel flies away with her prey, which never had a chance once she spotted it."

The family looked at our pretty kestrel female with respectful eyes.

"That's some bird!" said the older boy. "She doesn't look that fierce."

"I'll tell you another story. She came in with a male. For a while, they seemed to be getting along just fine. Then on Christmas Day, when we came in to feed the animals, we found that she had already had her dinner." I stopped and let them carry the story in their heads to its obvious conclusion.

"Do you mean SHE ate HIM?" gasped the mother.

"She did," I replied, "for Christmas dinner."

"I guess she is fierce," said the older boy.

"Are they around here?" asked the older girl with some apprehension.

"Oh, yes, although they are more common farther south. If you drive down the highway, you will see them sitting on fence wires every now and then. They are easy to identify if you look at their heads. Both the male and female have the dark cheek streak."

I moved along the trail. "This next cage has our hero in it. He is the Center's best known bird. He is a great horned owl, and his name is Orson. He can't be released because he has only one wing, but we keep him for educational purposes, and he goes to programs all over the state. He has probably been in more schools than all of you together!"

"Do all the animals have names?" asked the girl.

"All the permanent residents do. They are the ones who go out on programs, and when we bring a bird out, the first thing the children want to know is 'What's its name?' Only after they have been properly introduced will they listen to what we have to say about him. But we are careful NOT to name our patients. We have to remember that they are NOT pets. Remember the little fawns? They don't have names. The baby owls don't have names. Only the program birds are named."

"Why does he only have one wing? What happened to the other one?" asked the smaller boy.

THE SKUNKED OWL: ORSON'S STORY

The great horned owl sat on his favorite limb in his favorite tree and surveyed what he could of his territory. He seemed almost asleep. His eyes were half-closed, but his super-sensitive ears were hunting. The circular facial disc that made up his "face" acted like a satellite dish does for television waves. It collected and focused sounds to his ears which were positioned just like yours, on either side of his face. Unlike yours, however, one ear was slightly up and the other slightly down, so that he could not only identify sound, but could tell exactly where it was coming from. Suddenly his big yellow eyes opened wide, his huge wings spread as he left the branch in a dive to kill. His prey had no warning. The great wings were made of softly fringed feathers which let air escape and silenced any flapping sound. The owl was truly a "silent hunter of the night."

The owl's prey was a skunk, one of his favorites. The owl was sure of himself. He had a ninety-nine percent kill rate. He rarely missed. But there is always a first time. A branch deflected his attack. To protect his eyes, the nictitating membrane spread over the eye, obstructing his vision. His talons grasped the skunk, but it was not a clean kill. The skunk had a chance to twist around and bite sharply underneath the owl's wing, tearing muscle and membrane, before the talons re-gripped and contracted strongly for the kill.

Severely damaged, the hungry owl consumed part of the skunk before he tried unsuccessfully to fly. He tried again. One wing just did not work. He flopped frantically around on the forest floor, trying to get off the ground. Finally, exhausted, he came to rest near his prey, now having become vulnerable to predation himself.

The night passed and morning came. Still the owl was helpless. His wounds were dirty and becoming infected. But he still had

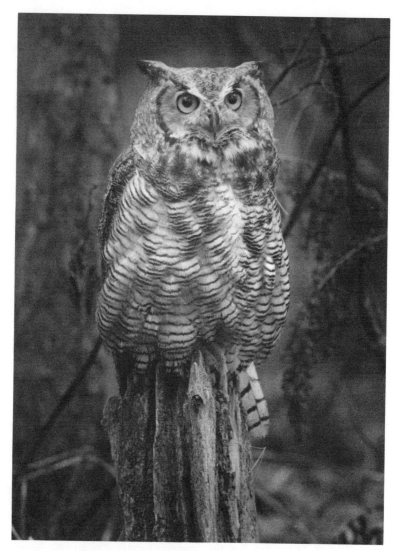

Orson poses behind the Center.

food. The day passed and a second night came with its dangers. The owl was in shock and severely stressed. He had lost a lot of blood. The wounds attracted flies, and by the next morning maggots were hatching. The owl survived another day, but was breathing heavily. He lay still and gave up the struggle.

So he was found on the forest floor, still as death, by some hikers enjoying the fine fall weather. One man wrapped the owl in his jacket and the group brought it to the Wildlife Hospital.

"Don't tell me," said Mark coming out of his office. "It's a great horned owl!"

"How did you know?" asked one of the hikers wonderingly.

"Smelled him," answered Mark, grinning. "Every great horned owl that is brought in for treatment smells like a skunk. They can't smell it but everybody else can! Let's have a look at him."

Mark took the owl to the back room and laid him on the counter that served as an examination table. As he spread the great left wing, he groaned. "This looks bad. We may not save him. First he needs some fluids and stimulants."

Mark took some change out of his pocket and went out the door. He came back with a can of Coca Cola. He poured some in a cup and boiled it in a microwave to get rid of the carbonation. Carefully, he inserted the feeding tube down the owl's throat. "C'mon, Fella, down she goes," he murmured encouragingly to the nearly dead owl. When the tube was in place, he handed the prepared bird to Dave and filled a syringe with the cooled boiled Coke. Slowly, he pushed the plunger and got the Coke on the inside. Ringer's solution was injected subcutaneously to give the bird more fluids. The dirty, infected wounds were cleaned gently, and the owl was given antibiotics. The great horned owl, fiercest of all the owls, was laid on his side in a cage, his eyes closed, his breathing shallow.

"Now, we wait," said Mark. "He may come around. He may not. Nothing more we can do." Mark took a long swallow out of the owl's Coke can.

"Give us a call tomorrow," he told the hikers. "We'll be better able to tell you how he's doing. Don't call too early. This is going to take awhile." The hikers left.

"What do you think?" Dave asked.

"I think we are going to have to put him down. He'll never fly again. Wing's too bad."

"Why wait?" asked Dave. "What's the point?"

"No point," answered Mark, who hated to put any animal down, especially owls. "But we'll just wait."

The following day, the owl was slightly improved. He received more fluids, more antibiotics, and the wounds were dressed again fresh and clean. But he did not eat, and he lay on the cage floor, both bad signs. Marty Smith had a look at him and agreed with Mark. The owl would never fly again, and probably should be put down. Still, Mark waited.

The next day, after treatment, the owl perched, a good sign, and later in the afternoon was force fed several ounces of mouse which he retained. But the bad wing drooped and all was definitely not well.

T.J. Dunn came over from the vet hospital and looked the owl over. "That's never going to heal. We'll have to amputate if we are going to save him. Those tissues are not getting blood. They are dying. That wing will kill him if we don't take it off."

Mark looked glum. "He's gone through a lot. Will he get through an amputation?"

"Maybe. Maybe not. But we'll never know till we try. If he dies under anesthesia, it's no worse than if we had to put him down." T.J. looked at the bird. "Let's give him a chance."

The operation was set for the first thing the next morning before the wildlife hospital or the vet hospital opened. The owl was

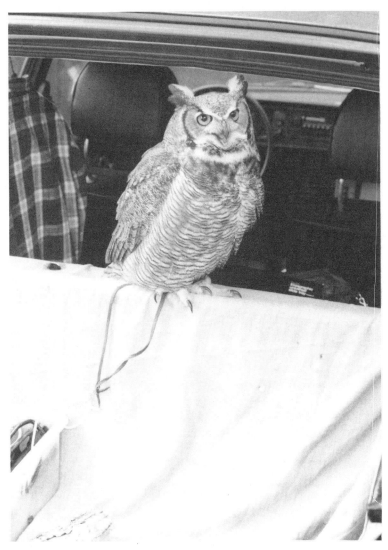

Orson, a Great Horned Owl, on the tailgate of his transportation to a program.

separated from his useless wing by the time the first dog owner brought his puppy in for shots. He lay on the cage floor recovering.

"Now, he can never be released," Dave said. "Now what happens? Our permit says we have to euthanize any bird we can't put back into the wild. You can't release a one-winged owl!"

Mark thought for a bit. "I think we are about to go more seriously into education. I think we need some birds on display for educational purposes, don't you?"

Dave stared for a minute and then smiled broadly. "Starting with a one-winged great horned owl? Yes!"

"Absolutely," answered Mark happily. "I think we should call him 'Orson'."

"Orson? Why Orson?"

"He looks like an 'Orson'," Mark said. "Let's write for the permit."

Orson recovered and had a long convalescence in an outside cage. He had a favorite perch from which he could see most of the outside activity, and on which his dinner was placed daily. Mark and Dave worked with him tirelessly to get him accustomed to people, and to teach him to sit on the fist to be shown off. The process was slow since Mark and Dave did not want him to be over-stressed. Orson never became tame, but he learned to tolerate being handled, and being shown.

At this writing, Orson has traveled over five thousand miles in the state of Wisconsin, and has appeared in hundreds of schools, camps, clubs, and civic organizations. He has attended a banquet and appeared on TV. He is not a wild bird living his normal life in the woods, but he has taught thousands of people about owls, about the woods, and about the care and treatment of wild animals and about the place of wildlife in our environment. He has accomplished a great deal of good in his life, all because Mark loved owls and wouldn't put him down.

"If you will come this way, I can show you Clawdia, our Bald Eagle. Look through this window. Oh, we're lucky. She is on her stump." Clawdia was sitting fairly close to the window and did indeed look impressive. The family stared in silence for a few moments.

"That's the first eagle I've ever seen that close. They are huge, aren't they?" said the mother.

"What IS the wing span? Five feet or so?" asked the father.

"Closer to six or seven feet. She is about three feet tall and weighs nine pounds," I said.

"Seems like she should weigh more than that," commented the father. "She's a big bird."

"Yes, but there are a lot of feathers there and feathers are practically weightless. Her actual body is not all that big. You see her white head and her white tail? That means she is a grownup eagle. Can you guess how old she is?"

The smaller boy said, "Fifty years old?"

"No, not that old."

"Twenty?" guessed the girl.

"No." I looked at the smaller boy. "How old are you?"

"Eight," he said proudly.

"Well, what do you know? That's just how old Clawdia is!"

"You said she was a grownup." He looked at me accusingly.

"She is, for an eagle. When a bald eagle is a baby, it is all brown, and some people mistake it for a hawk or maybe a golden eagle because it doesn't have the white head we think of when we think 'bald eagle'. But it doesn't get that until it is five or six years old.

Then, when the head and tail are white and the beak and feet are yellow, it is a grown-up eagle and can mate and have baby eagles."

"I heard they mate for life. Is that true?" asked the father.

"Yes, it's true. In the wild, anything can happen. Man is the greatest predator. Even though it is illegal to shoot a bird of prey, and certainly illegal to shoot an eagle, which is just recently off the endangered list, we have not had one eagle in here that hasn't shown shotgun pellets in an X-ray. It may have come in for something quite different, but the pellets are there when we look."

"That's awful!" said the mother. "Who would do that?"

"Who knows?" I shrugged. "No one would ever admit it. The fine is too steep. But around here we don't feel a bit friendly toward anyone who would be so trigger happy as to shoot an eagle."

"Was she shot?"

"No. This bird came in as a baby. Nobody had a chance to shoot her. She came from the Koller Cranberry Marsh in Manitowish Waters.

THE CRANBERRY EAGLE

Shortly after the Center opened, the phone rang, and I grabbed for it. I played a little game with myself always trying to catch it before the second ring. I was not always successful, but it was a small triumph when I did.

"Northwoods Wildlife Center. This is Sybil. May I help you?"

The voice on the other end was deep and rough. "This is the Koller Cranberry Marsh. We've got a baby eagle here that can't fly. Can you do something about it?"

"Where are you?" I asked. He told me, and since this was before we were given a truck, my station wagon served the purpose. Dave loaded the big musky net into the back, plus an animal carrier borrowed from Foster-Smith. He added a pair of welder's gloves, and we were ready.

When we got to the marsh, the foreman showed us where he had last seen the baby. Please remember that I was very new at this bird ambulance business. When I heard "baby" I had visions of a small handful of fluffy feathers. I was certainly not prepared for the giant bird lumbering around the edges of a cranberry marsh. "Baby" indeed. He was a HORSE! He was at least a yard tall and when he tried to fly, his wing span was awesome. He didn't even look like an eagle. He was brown. No white head. No white tail. "Is that it?" I asked Dave, unbelievingly.

"That's it," he answered. "Now to catch him. You go around and start him toward me. I'll net him."

I walked around the marsh pond until I was facing the eaglet. It was pretty obvious that he didn't like being cornered. I was moving, though, and Dave was still. He turned away from me and headed toward Dave. No matter what you might have heard

161

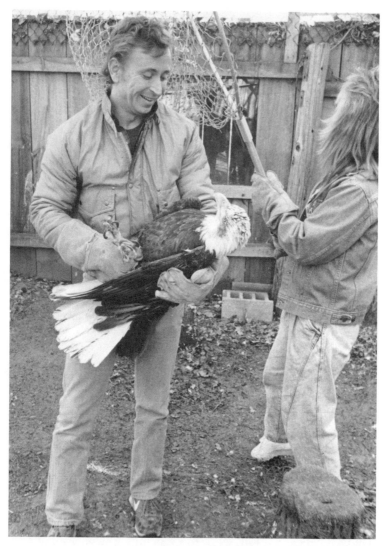

Dave with the new "Clawdia," who is in the midst of getting her adult plumage. Volunteer Janis Schneider holds the net.

about the graceful majesty of a soaring eagle, there is nothing graceful about a walking one. This eagle waddled with a kind of ungainly rolling gait that no one would ever write poetry about. As he gained speed he hunched his wings, spread them, and thereby doubled in size. Dave had the net ready. He suddenly jumped up right in front of the bird and brought the net down over him. A successful capture.

Naturally the eagle did not take quietly to being netted, and soon managed to struggle himself into a tangle of net, feathers and talons, all of which eventually had to be separated, with everything belonging to the eagle being stuffed into the carrier, and the net, or what was left of it, stowed back in the car.

Since Dave had the welder's gloves, he worked on the talons, trying to free their grasp on the net. As he released one grip the eagle reached frantically for another. The actual capture took less than five minutes. The rest of the hour was spent peeling the net off the eagle and making him let go of the mesh. Dave was relatively new at this game, too. It didn't help that we had an audience of cranberry workers cheering us on. As Dave released each section of net, I would pull it away, and finally Dave had the eagle in his arms. He held it in the "football carry" where the bird lay cradled in his arms on its back, with Dave's gloved hand holding the feet securely. I carried the net and we walked back to the car. We stood for a moment contemplating the door of the animal carrier, and measuring it against the now quiet eagle. I could see Dave struggling with a decision.

"I'll hold him on my lap," he announced at length.

I opened the passenger side door and he climbed inside. The eagle lay absolutely still — not a wiggle. I closed the door and went around to my side. I started the motor. The eagle never flicked an eye. He acted as if he had ridden around in cars for twenty years and found it dull. The ride, however, was anything but dull for Dave and me. At any moment, the eagle could struggle for release or use his strong hooked beak and talons. A fighting eagle in the front seat of a car was anything but safe for traffic. But it didn't happen. The eagle behaved, and we made it back to the Center without incident.

Mark met us at the door. He and Dave examined the baby eagle in the back room, but could find no overt injuries. They X-rayed both wings and found nothing.

"Maybe he is younger than the others in the nest. Maybe he just needs a little more time," Mark said. "Let's see what a week or two of growing will do." This time, Mark was cradling the eagle and took him into the flight room and gently released him.

The eagle ran clumsily to the far end of the room and turned to face Mark. Glaring, he shook out his rumpled feathers, and flapped his wings to straighten everything out. When he felt himself again, he explored his new territory with that same awkward rolling gait. Obviously, talons were not made for walking. Since he could not fly to the perches in the flight room, Mark put a log on the floor for him to sit on. Next, he added a large, shallow tub of water for bathing and drinking, and a couple of rats for dinner. Granted, he was a captured bird, but his accommodations were deluxe.

He stayed with us for two weeks. Somehow, in that period, "he" became "she" just because of the way she looked and acted. We had no way of "sexing" her for sure, but Mark was an expert on birds, and his opinion carried weight. Her size and configuration told him that she was a female.

Meanwhile, we had applied to the U.S. Fish and Wildlife Service for a permit to have a resident eagle. One was waiting for us at the University of Minnesota Raptor Center, ready to be shipped as soon as our permit was granted. Mark watched the mail every day, eager for the permit to arrive. He really wanted a captive disabled eagle to show at the Center for educational purposes. Eagles were endangered and many people had never seen one close-up. It was a golden opportunity, not only to show what the majestic bird looked like, but to talk about why it was endangered and what people could do to help bring it back.

When the cranberry bird's two weeks were up, it was time to take her back to the marsh and release her. If we had been right, she would have developed enough to fly by now and take her place in the wild population. We called Koller Marsh and told them we were coming. This time the eagle traveled in the carrier. We took the net along, "Just in case...."

Our telephone call was a clarion cry all over the marsh. The whole crew gathered to see the baby eagle fly. Dave extricated her from the carrier with some difficulty, and carried her out to the same part of the marsh where we had picked her up. She would be familiar with the area and feel comfortable there.

Dave tested the wind. "I'll toss her up this way," he told me. "You stand over there and watch where she goes." He directed me to a slightly raised bank around the edge of the marsh where I would have a wide view of the area. I trudged around to the opposite side of the marsh.

"Ok!" I called back to Dave.

The crews stood silent, expectant. Dave held the bird in front of him with both arms extended. He set himself, bent his knees and gave a mighty heave. The bird rose, flapping her wings, and plunked down five feet away! Without stopping to think of dangerous talons or beak, Dave ran over and picked her up before she even had a chance to realize he was coming.

"Once more," he called.

"Ready," I answered.

Big as it is, an eagle weighs only about ten pounds. Most of the bulk is feathers, and those feather shafts are hollow. This time he gave her a mighty toss and the eagle sailed up into the air, flapping wildly, and this time crash landed about ten feet out! The workers were politely silent, but some of them had broad smiles on their faces. Dave's face was red.

"Guess she needs more time," he said.

This time the eagle was not about to be caught by hand. Dave went back to the car for the net while I watched to see where she went. She stayed where she had landed, recovering from her alarming excursions into the air. But when she saw Dave with the net, she bolted, running and flapping as fast as she could. Dave had to run to catch up with her and get in position to net her. The crews thought this was just as entertaining as the abortive flights. Finally, Dave was successful, and again we went through the process of extricating a determined eagle from the net. After much work and little progress, he picked up eagle and net together and put both into the car.

"Let's go," he said.

Back at the Center, Mark and Dave both worked to separate talons and net, and released the bird back into the flight room.

"There's got to be a reason," said Mark. "We didn't find anything. Let's ship her over to the Raptor Center and let them look her over."

"Good idea," agreed Dave, who had had his fill of baby eagles for a while.

The mail came bringing our eagle permit! We rejoiced and called the Raptor Center. "We'll trade you," said Mark to Pat Redig, the director. "We'll send you our bird that we can't find anything wrong with, and you can send over our captive eagle."

That is how the Koller eagle left Rhinelander airport in the morning, and in the afternoon, the plane returned with our very own resident eagle. The new bird was also a juvenile, but had a permanently disabled wing. It was older than the Koller bird. It would have its adult plumage in a year or so. This bird had been handled and trained to the fist. Both Dave and Mark could carry it for short distances only a few days after it arrived. It was a perfect education bird.

We had a contest, announced in our newsletter, to name the new eagle. We had intended the contest for children, but the idea

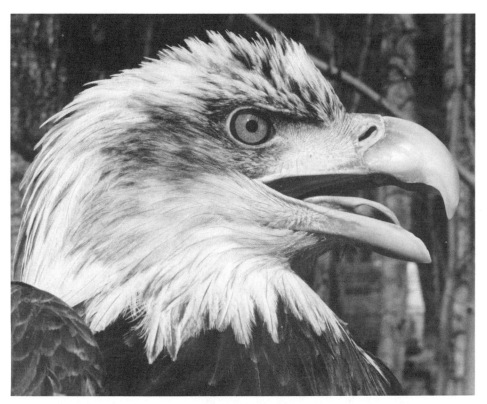

Clawdia II has matured into her adult plumage, including the characteristic white head of a bald eagle. When she was first picked up in the cranberry Marsh, she was just a baby. At the time of this writing, she is nearly eight years old.

seemed to appeal to all ages, and many people sent in names for the bird, a female. "Miss Liberty," "Miss America" and "Freedom" dominated the list, none of which appealed to us. Then a ten-year-old girl in Milwaukee sent in "Clawdia," and we all pounced. "That's it! That's her name!" The little girl won a T-shirt and our eagle had a name.

After examination, the Raptor Center announced that the cranberry eagle had a separated shoulder and would probably never fly because the position of the injury rendered it inoperable.

We heard the news with regret and notified the Koller people, and that, we thought, would be the last we heard of the cranberry eagle.

A year went by. Many visitors saw and heard about Clawdia. She became a celebrity, even being on television every now and then, doing her part for the Center and for the cause of eagles in Wisconsin. But she continued to live in her cage until one day we had a call from another rehabilitator who wanted to work with her and extend her training. After much deliberation and much telephoning, we received permission to lend the bird, and the man picked her up to school her. He did indeed school her. He took her to schools on programs. Our bird, who had spent her life in safety in her cage was suddenly subject to stresses that she was unprepared and unable to handle. The man may not have realized what he was putting her through, or he may just have been enjoying the effect he created by carrying a live eagle around in public. For whatever reason, the bird was ill when she was brought back and never recovered from the experience. Shortly thereafter she died of stress-induced visceral gout. There was nothing we could do. Even the Raptor Center was helpless. Clawdia died and we mourned with the usual "if only..."

We called the Raptor Center. We still had the permit. Would they trust us with another eagle? They would. It would arrive the following day on the afternoon plane. Mark and Dave met the plane. By this time we had been given a big, red pickup truck and I was no longer the pickup car.

The new eagle was also a female. We named her Clawdia II and put her in the new eagle cage just outside the window of the Center's reception room. All her papers had accompanied her, but it was a while before we even cared where she came from because we were so busy installing her properly in the Center. When Dave sat down to look at the papers, he yelled, running into Mark's tiny office. "This is our eagle! Look! It's a copy of the chart we sent over with her. She's ours!"

And so she was. The cranberry eagle had come home. She still lives at the Center and may be seen any day during visitors' hours.

But we've never tried to school her, and she isn't very fond of Dave for some reason.

Clawdia left her stump and, spreading her huge wings, flapped herself up to the far perch.

"She is doing much better since she has matured. When she first came she would fly from the high perch to the low perch and then to the stump. It took her a long time to decide to fly back. She would go from one foot to the other and eye the next perch. You could almost see her psyching herself up for the big try. Then she would take off and land on the lower perch and go through the same performance, while she planned her flight to the high perch. It was almost as if she were deliberately practicing her flying. Now, since she has matured, for some reason she is much better at it. She will take off from the high perch and fly in a big circle all around the cage and land wherever she pleases. It doesn't seem to take as much effort," I explained.

"If she can fly, can't she be released?" asked the girl.

"I'm afraid not. She has been with us for eight years and would not know how to care for herself in the wild. Her parents never taught her how to fish. For eight years, all the local fisherman have been bringing her presents. She doesn't know how to fish for herself."

"Couldn't you teach her?" asked the smaller boy.

"How?" I challenged him. "I can't fly. I can't dive for fish. She needs her parents to show her how. She will have to stay here. Anyway, her shoulder isn't really well. She is just flying better now. She has a long way to go, really."

"Will she stay here?"

"Yes, and do you know what we are hoping?"

"What?"

"We are hoping she will be a foster mother to baby eagles that are brought in. We have had a couple of babies this year that we put in that cage right next to Clawdia's cage so that they could see her and watch her fly. But we want to be able to make a nest and let Clawdia take care of the babies right in that cage. Orson, the great-horned owl, takes care of all of our great-horned owl babies, and Bart, the barred owl, has raised barred owl babies. There is no reason that Clawdia couldn't be a foster mother to eaglets if she were asked."

"How does it happen that you get baby eagles?" asked the mother.

"That's interesting. The Department of Natural Resources watches all the known eagle nests very carefully every spring and checks to see how many eggs are in each nest. They make a list of which nest has how many eggs, and later in the season, they rearrange things so that each nest gets two eaglets."

"That's weird. Do they steal the eggs?"

"No, it makes good sense. A pair of eagles can hunt well enough to supply two babies with ample food. The third eaglet in a nest comes out on the short end of the stick. He is the last to hatch. Since baby eagles grow from three inches to three feet in three months, his siblings grow so fast that even the two or three days between the first to hatch and the third make a big difference in size. The little guy gets pushed aside by his bigger siblings and doesn't get his head up high enough to get the food. He usually starves, maybe gets pushed out of the nest entirely or, if he does survive, is a runt and malnourished. The DNR people take the number three eaglet out of the nest and put it in a nest where there is one other eaglet of about the same size. The parents adopt the new baby and everything is fine. All the eaglets have a chance to grow up. Sometimes, while a foster nest is being decided upon, we get the extra babies to care for. Clawdia could help us there. If Clawdia is taking care of them, the baby eagles would not be imprinted. An eagle would be feeding them."

"Is Clawdia imprinted?"

"No, her parents raised her until she was ready to fly. She knows she's an eagle."

"How long will she live?" asked the mother.

"In captivity, fifty years is not unheard of. In the wild she would not live that long. Eagles have territorial fights and sometimes damage each other seriously. They also have man to contend with. They get shot, hit by cars, they run into windows and powerlines, get tangled in fishing lines, caught in traps, poisoned — any number of things can happen to shorten their natural lives."

"How do you know she's a girl?" the girl wanted to know.

"We don't, really," I replied. "We are just guessing. Eagles, hawks, owls, swans, loons and many other birds have the same plumage for both the males and females. You can only know for sure if you operate on them and look inside. It doesn't really matter to us. So we just name them and hope we are right."

"What if you're wrong?" asked the older boy.

"We just change the name."

"But how do you know you are wrong?" he persisted.

"The females lay eggs when they are mature. Ascha, our red-tailed hawk is definitely a girl. She made a nest and laid eggs early in the spring. We know she's a she."

"Where is she?" asked the small boy. "Can we see her?"

"If you'll look in the cage across the trail, you will see Ascha. She is imprinted."

The family crossed over to the opposite window and looked into Ascha's cage. She was sitting on a tree limb facing the trail. Her white belly was very visible.

"This is a red-tailed hawk, but all you can see right now is her tummy. If she turns around, you will be able to see her red tail. Actually, it's a bronzy red, but it is beautiful when the sun shines on it."

"She certainly has a fat tummy!" exclaimed the mother.

"Right now, she probably weighs a lot more grams than she should. There is nothing wrong with her physically. She is one of the imprinted birds. She belonged to a falconer, and he imprinted her on purpose so that she would work with him and hunt for him. He had to leave her with us when he moved to Alaska because he could not take her with him. As you can see, there is nothing wrong with her flight!" Ascha had just swooped around her big flight cage and landed in another tree. "There, look! Now you can see her tail."

"Oh, it is red! What a lovely bird!" exclaimed the mother.

"It looks brown to me." said the smaller boy.

"It's red, like some people's hair is red," explained his father.

"But that's not REALLY red," complained the boy. "Not really, really RED!" he said.

"Well, no. I guess not. But it's red-tailed hawk red. How about that?" smiled his father.

"Ok, I guess," conceded the boy. "But not really red."

"Ascha is a very good hunter. Any chipmunk or mouse that ventures into her cage quickly becomes dinner. I've even see her catch and kill a grass snake. But we can't know that she is going to catch something for herself, so we feed her every day. She gets pretty tubby in the summer when there is lots of dinner running around in her cage. In the winter, she thins down."

"Does she stay out here all winter?" asked the girl.

"Yes. So long as she has plenty of food, she gets along just fine. In the wild, she would probably migrate to follow her food supply. In the fall, there's a great place to see hawks. It is called Hawk Ridge. It's near Duluth, Minnesota. It's on what is called the Mississippi flyway where the hawks fly around Lake Superior and down the Mississippi. For some reason, they don't like to fly across the lake. Thousands and thousands of different kinds of hawks can be seen there in the fall. Probably the second week in September is best. It depends on the weather. If you have a chance, go and see them. It is a real experience."

"We live near St. Paul. It wouldn't be a bad trip. Maybe we'll try it this fall," said the father. "Hawk Ridge, you say?"

"Yes. Take your binoculars. There'll be lots of birders there. Biologists will be banding them. You can see mist nets at work. It's fascinating. The birds are caught, but not injured. Then they get little bands on their ankles with numbers. The numbers are recorded and the birds are released to continue their journey. If you ever find a dead bird with a band on its ankle, you take off the band and send it to the US Fish and Wildlife Service with a note about where you found it and how you happened to find the bird. Then the USFWS can look in their books to see where they banded that bird and write down what happened to it."

"There's a lot more to birds than I thought," said the older boy. "I never saw a bird with an ankle bracelet on."

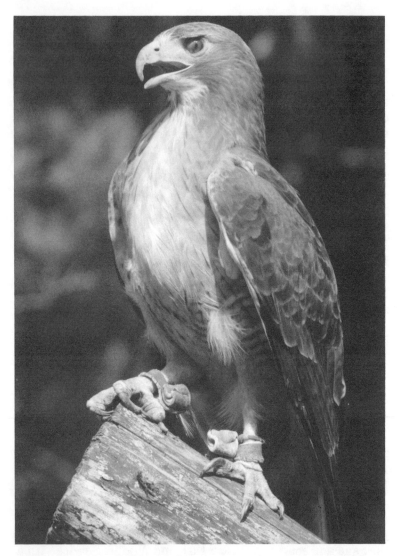

Ascha, the red-tailed hawk, has straps, or jesses, on her ankles so that she can be held on the fist.

"We had a banded owl brought into the Center one day. He had been hit by a car, but the only thing that had been hurt was his tail. All the feathers were broken or gone. Otherwise, he was fine. When that happens, what you do is 'imp' or implant some feathers in the broken shafts, and then you don't have to hold the bird through a whole molting period while he grows his own. When he molts, he loses the implanted feathers and grows his own naturally. Soon, he is as good as new. Meanwhile he can be out in the wild, which is a definite plus."

"Did you 'imp' his feathers?" asked the smaller boy.

"That's exactly what we did," I replied. "But there was a little problem."

"What?"

"We hadn't been going very long and hadn't had a chance to collect lots of owl feathers. We just didn't have any owl tail feathers. You see, feathers are not all the same. Some fit on the right side and some fit on the left, and some belong in the tail. The only tail feathers we had belonged to a red-tailed hawk."

"Like Ascha?" asked the girl.

"Like Ascha," I agreed. "So we did the only thing we could do. We imped the hawk feathers into the owl!"

"How do you imp?" asked the older boy. "Do you glue them on?"

"Well, sort of. First you cut about a one-half to three-quarter-inch-long piece of split bamboo. It has to be small enough to fit into the feather shaft. Remember that bird's feather shafts are hollow. That's why they used to use feathers for writing. They would sharpen the end of the shaft into a point and dip it into the ink. The hollow shaft held the ink, and people wrote with 'quill pens'."

"What about imping?" demanded the smaller boy.

"Sorry, I got off the subject. Well, after you have the right number of bamboo pieces for the feathers you are going to implant, you trim the feathers left on the bird as short as possible without getting so short it might hurt. Then you glue the little bamboo pieces into the hollow ends you have left, letting half of the bamboo stick out of the shaft so that the new feathers can be put on. Next you trim the new feathers to the right length to fit the bird when they have been glued on."

"Do you really glue them?" asked the boy.

"Yes, with waterproof glue, so it won't dissolve if it gets wet."

"By now, the first pieces of bamboo are securely stuck in the feather shafts and you can glue the new feathers to them. You take the feathers in order. Remember they are not all alike. Then you glue the new feathers on the prepared shafts and the bird is as good as new."

"Does the bird let you do it?" asked the girl.

"He gets a tranquilizer, so he will lie quietly while you work on him. Otherwise, he would thrash around and you couldn't get the feathers right."

"Did you let the owl go?" asked the girl.

"Yes, but remember that owl had a hawk's tail. He could fly just fine, but he would have a hawk's tail until he molted, and molting time was several months away. Remember, too, that he was banded."

"What happened?" she asked.

"Well, that owl wasn't very smart. He had been hit by a car when he was first brought in, and several months later, just as molting began, he was hit by a car again! This time, he wasn't so lucky just to lose his tail. This time, he was killed. The man who hit him noticed the band and called the Department of Natural Resources. They asked him to bring the owl in. Can you imagine

176

what happened in the DNR office when a man brought in a dead barred owl with a red-tailed hawk's tail?"

"I'll bet they were surprised!" giggled the smaller boy.

"You bet right," I answered "until one man felt the tail and could feel the imping. Then they called us and we confessed that we had put him together once before."

"I'll bet that was something. A red-tailed owl," The older boy grinned. "I'll bet they didn't believe it."

The family stood a moment savoring the joke. "Do you have an owl tail now?" asked the smaller boy.

"Yes, we save all the molted feathers, and now we could do the job right."

"Do you have eagle feathers? Can I have one?" asked the smaller boy.

"Yes, we have some, and no, you can't have one. That's against the law. You'd be fined if you were caught with an eagle feather."

"Why?"

"Because you couldn't prove that you had not killed an eagle to get it."

"Even if I picked it up myself?"

"Even if you picked it up yourself. Even we are not allowed to keep any more eagle feathers than we might need for imping. All the rest are sent to the Fish and Wildlife Service. That department apportions eagle feathers among the different Indian tribes that apply for them for their ceremonies."

We moved down the trail from Ascha's cage.

"That is George, a short-eared owl. No, don't look up. George is a ground nester. He stays close to the ground. There he is in the corner under the bush. He's hiding."

"I see him!!" said the girl. "Oh, he's cute."

"What's wrong with him?" asked the mother.

"Another car strike. The owls hunt along the highway and just don't get out of the way in time."

"Is it his wing?" asked the father. "It seems to droop on the left there."

"Yes, his wing didn't heal right. When a break is near a joint, it is almost impossible to set it properly. It can't be pinned, because there is nothing to pin to. George had a shoulder injury. The break couldn't be pinned. Can you see his facial disk? See how the feathers grow around his beak? All owls look like they have a 'face'."

The children peered into George's cage at close range. The parents looked over their heads.

"Are those pointy things his short ears?" asked the girl.

"No, owls are described as 'horned' or 'long-eared' or 'short-eared' but those are only feather tufts. They have nothing to do with hearing."

"Doesn't he have any ears?" the smaller boy asked.

"Oh, yes, he has ears. They are on either side of his face, just the way yours are. His facial disk focuses the sounds to his ears. He can hear better than you can!"

"Aw.." said the smaller boy, disbelieving.

"He does most of his hunting with his ears. He sits in a tree and listens. He may even have his eyes closed, but he is hunting. He could hear a mouse running under the leaves or even under snow. He swoops down at it and bingo! Dinner! If there is snow, you can see where an owl has caught his dinner because there is a hole in the snow and a 'snow angel' wing mark around it where he took off with his prey. Watch for it if you are in the woods this winter."

"Do they ever miss?" asked the older boy.

"Not very often. Owls have a 99 percent kill rate. Hawks have an 85 to 88 percent kill rate. Owls are very efficient hunters. George, here, is a little different from most owls. He flies in the daytime. Most owls are nocturnal and fly at night. He also builds his own nest. Remember, I said owls rent a pre-owned nest the following year. But George, the short-eared owl, builds his own and builds it on the ground instead of in a tree."
"On the ground?" commented the father. "That's unusual."

"Yes, it's called a 'scrape'. He finds a protected place in the grass and scrapes a hole which he lines with grass and feathers and that's home."

"Now, if you will look behind you, you will meet Sadie, the screech owl. She is small, but she is full grown."

The whole family changed its focus and peered at Sadie.

"She's sleeping," said the mother.

"Well, it is daytime, and she usually is more active at night, but right now she is trying to con you into thinking she is an old, broken-off branch on a tree."

"Of course! You could walk right by and not really see her!"

The group all examined Sadie's picture on a plaque next to her cage that had the information about her.

"South Dakota! She's a long way from home," said the father. "Was she really a tourist attraction? How is that possible? I thought you couldn't keep an owl."

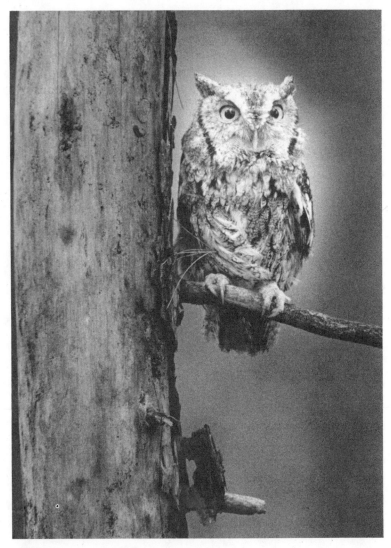

Sadie, the little screech owl, perches in the Center's flight room.

THE GAS STATION AD

I continued the tour. "If you look over here, you'll see Patti. She is a saw whet owl and smaller than Sadie. She would have to be very wary, too."

The family all looked for a few seconds in silence.

"She's darling!" exclaimed the girl. "Oh, can't I hold her?"

It was a storm to end all storms! The thunder rolled across the sky and exploded over the little gas station alongside the highway. Emmy was terrified of storms, but there were customers sheltering in the store part of the station, and she couldn't curl herself up in a ball in her favorite chair and shut her eyes and hold her ears till Tim shook her and said it was all right now. As each thunderclap resounded through the clouds, she cowered and hunched her shoulders a little tighter. Would it never stop? Tim came in from pumping gas and wiped his dripping face and hair with a couple of paper towels from the rest room. He shook the rain off his jacket on the rough wood floor.

The station was built of logs in the tradition of the pioneers that had come in covered wagons across South Dakota along the same trail before it was a US highway. It was heated by a wood stove in winter, and cooled by the breeze, if there was one, in the blazing summers. Behind the station and store were the living quarters. They couldn't actually be called a "house", but until something better came along, it was what they had. Tim and Emmy had operated the station for twenty-two years, waiting for something better to come along. It hadn't. They were almost resigned to that fact. But hope does not easily die. "You never know," said Tim, "what's going to happen tomorrow, don't you know."

"You can't tell until it happens," was Emmy's reply.

At last the storm passed its rumbling way to the east, and as the clouds traveled with it, the sun blinked out from behind the last one. Steam started rising from the sodden earth, and the smell of soil and growing things wafted into the now-open door. The waiting customers left to continue their journeys, and Emmy and Tim were alone.

"Believe I'll look around," said Tim. "OK with you?"

"Fine," answered Emmy. "I'll just stand here in the door and smell the spring."

She was standing there when the car drove up. The driver rolled the window down and called out? "I gotta baby bird in my hat. It's soaking wet. Can you do anything for it? I can't do any good driving."

"Sure," said Emmy. "We can take care of it. We've raised a lot of 'em." She approached the car. The man offered her his hat.

"Here, take it. You can take the hat, too. It's no good now, anyway."

Emmy took the hat into her hands and inspected the contents. There was a small, very sodden bird sitting miserably inside. It's eyes were closed, and it was very still.

"You want gas?" asked Emmy.

"No, don't need it. I was just looking for a place to leave the bird. Sorry."

"That's OK. I'll just take the bird inside then."

"Thanks," said the man. "So long." He put the car into gear and took off down the highway.

Emmy took the bird out of the hat and held it in her warm hands. The tiny cold feet clutched her fingers. She looked at it more carefully. "You're an owl!" she told it, surprised. "I didn't know you would be an owl." She smiled and went back into the store.

She tried to towel the bird dry, but that just plastered the feathers to the body. She put it into a small box and went to get her hair dryer. When her arm got tired, she propped the dryer on some cereal boxes and just moved the bird around under it. Slowly the feathery down dried. The tiny owl stood up several times and stretched and shook his minute wings. He was coming around.

Tim came back and looked at her in some surprise. "Where'd you find that?" he asked.

"Fellow stopped and gave it to me. Had it in his hat."

"Must have got washed out of its nest. Or the whole nest went. Did he say how he got it?"

"I guess I never asked. Emmy shrugged. "It don't matter. The bird is here now. It's an owl."

"An owl?"

"Sure. Look at its face. And its eyes."

"Guess you're right. Looks like an owl. What kind?"

"I don't know. Wait until it gets a little bigger."

A car drove up to the station and Tim started out the door. "What you going to feed it?" he asked and disappeared.

Emmy stood pondering. That was going to be a problem. Then she smiled. She called all of her three neighbors and asked them to start setting mouse traps. "I got a baby owl to feed," she explained proudly. Life was definitely getting interesting.

Emmy fed the baby, and it thrived. It grew its flight feathers and learned to fly in its new home. Emmy was afraid to let it outside for fear it would fly away, and she didn't want to lose her baby.

Her neighbor to the west, Earl Evenson, came by one day with a couple of mice. He always liked to visit with the little owl. If you fed the animal, you got a kind of proprietary feeling about it. It was HIS owl, too. "Hi, Buttons," he greeted it. "Looks like you ain't ever going to grow."

Emmy bridled immediately. "He'll grow in his own time, Earl." she said. "Maybe his kind of owl doesn't grow as fast as others."

"Calm down, Emmy. I didn't mean nothing. It's just he ain't getting any bigger. You can see that."

Emmy relaxed. "I guess I can," she admitted. "I just hope he's all right. I'd sure hate to lose him after all this time."

"He seems healthy. You know, you'd ought to show him off to people. Ain't many people ever seen an owl close up. You should have a sign out on the highway. 'Stop and see a real owl. People would stop to see it and they'd buy gas maybe, or a Coke."

Emmy stared. "That's a great idea. I never thought of that."

Tim came in from pumping gas and joined the conversation as he made change. He was visibly excited about the idea. When the car had driven off, he came back with a wide smile on his face. "Maybe this owl will make the difference. Maybe this is what we've needed, don't you know." He hugged Emmy, and she leaned against him.

So it was that the sign went up. "STOP IN AND SEE OUR LIVE OWL. BUY GAS AND SHOP WHILE YOU LOOK. BAILEY'S GENERAL STORE. TWO MILES."

It worked. People did stop to see Buttons, so named for his two bright yellow eyes. Buttons flew around the store, perched on the canned tomatoes or the bags of coffee beans waiting to go through the grinder. He was wary enough to stay just out of reach, but he was a great show, and business flourished. Emmy took to feeding him hamburger so people could watch him eat. She was reluctant to feed him mouse where anyone could see.

Earl stopped by, even if his mice were no longer needed. He really liked Buttons. "You want me to clip his wings like I do my chickens?" he asked one day. "He couldn't fly then, and you wouldn't have to worry about him getting out the door when people leave."

"Seems like a good idea," Tim said.

"I don't know," said Emmy. "Won't it hurt him?"

"No more'n cutting your nails," said Earl. "One snip each wing and it's done. Nothing to it."

"Well, all right. You go ahead. Maybe that would be better," Emmy agreed.

"I'll be over tomorrow. About this time. Maybe later," Earl promised and left.

The next day, Earl arrived with his clippers. The next step was to catch Buttons, who suddenly felt skittish about being caught. The three people grabbed as he flew frantically about the store. No matter where he flew, there was a human there to pounce at him. He grew careless in his terror and crashed into the tall rolling ladder with which items were obtained from the top shelves. He dropped to the floor and lay still.

"Oh! He's dead! He's killed," Emmy wailed, and ran to pick up the small ball of inert feathers from the floor.

"Here, I can clip him now," said Earl. "He won't even know what happened."

"No! No! Leave him alone. Oh, he's dead. I know he's dead!"

"Feel his chest. Listen if his heart is beating. Maybe he ain't dead after all," Tim said. "Here, let me listen." Tim reached for Buttons.

"No! I'll listen. Everybody keep quiet." Emmy lowered her head to the bird's chest. The quiet was ominous. Suddenly, she looked up. "It is!" it's beating. He's not dead. I knew he couldn't be dead!" she contradicted herself. "I knew it." She burst into tears and cried all over the still unconscious bird.

"Let be." Tim consoled her. "There, there, now. It'll be all right now, don't you know."

Emmy sniffed and became calmer. "But he's not going to get clipped. That's what started this. I know you meant no harm, but no thanks."

Earl shrugged. "Just trying to help," he said uncomfortably. "Guess I'd better be going." He escaped.

Slowly Buttons began to recover. Soon, he perched on Emmy's shoulder, but one wing had been damaged. He might as well have been clipped. The wing did not improve, and Buttons could no longer fly. He fluttered, he climbed with beak and feet, but his days of flying around the station were over.

Two miles down the highway, two men had gotten out of their car and were taking pictures of the "See the live owl" sign. "Do you suppose that's for real?" asked one.

"They wouldn't advertise it that way if it weren't.

"Don't they know they're in trouble?"

"Probably not, or they wouldn't do it. Let's go."

The men got back into the car and drove to the 'live owl gas station.' On the side of the car was the insignia "US Fish and Wildlife Service." Tim saw it as he went out to pump gas.

"No gas," said the driver. "We came to see the owl."

"Oh, sure. Come on in the station. He's in there. We call him Buttons." Tim led the way. Maybe they didn't want gas, but his experience told him that they would buy something, once they got in and saw the owl. Everybody did. It was a real good ad.

"Emmy. Couple fellows want to see Buttons."

"Come in. He's right over here on the back counter. See him?"

"A little screech," said one man.

"He just didn't seem to grow very big. I'll get some hamburger if you'd like to see him eat," Emmy offered, and turned to the cooler.

"Looks like the gray phase. Something's wrong with his wing. See, the left one. It hangs a bit."

Emmy returned with a small wad of hamburger. "Yes, he's got a bad wing. He had an accident. He flew into the ladder."

"Oh?" asked one of the men. "How did that happen? Never mind feeding it."

Emmy gave Buttons a bite of hamburger. "We were trying to catch him to clip his wings so he couldn't fly out the door," she explained. "He kept wanting to fly outside, and we were afraid he'd get away. Earl, our neighbor was going to clip him, but he hit the ladder."

The man who had been driving took a deep breath. "Why didn't you just let him fly away?"

"Oh, we couldn't do that," said Tim, smiling. "Emmy saved him after a storm. He kinda got to be our owl. He helps the business, too. People stop by to see him, just like you," He added hopefully. "Then maybe they buy a little something."

"Sorry," said the other man. "We're US Fish and Wildlife. It's illegal to keep a bird of prey. We'll have to take him with us."

"NO!" cried Emmy. "Not Buttons." She dived for the owl and rushed into the back rooms.

"Sorry, Mister. But that's our job. You're breaking the law keeping the owl. Not only that, but you aren't feeding it right, and you are using it for commercial purposes. Ignorance of the law is not a valid excuse. I shall have to issue a citation, and you will have to appear in court. Now, go and talk to you wife." The man was pleasant, but firm, and after a pause, Tim went. The driver wrote the citation, and laid it on the counter.

Emmy did not return, but they could hear her sobs. Tim brought the owl out in his hands.

"Guess you need a box," he said quietly.

"No, that's not necessary. We always carry a container in the car." The man took the owl. "I'm sorry about your wife," he said and turned to the door.

The driver followed. Then he turned back. "Give us a coupla Cokes and a bag of potato chips." He took out his wallet. "Keep the change," he said, and left.

Back in the car, he turned to his partner. "Why do I always feel so awful? We are doing the right thing, but I feel like a skunk."

"But they weren't doing the right thing. This bird is malnourished, permanently injured, and who knows what else. They should feel like skunks, not you."

"That's true," agreed the driver, "but I don't feel any better."

Within a week, a small screech owl arrived at the Wildlife Center to take up residence as an education bird. Since no one had thought to include the name on the records that arrived with the bird, 'Buttons' became 'Sadie' and bears that name today. No one knows for sure whether the little owl is a male or female, since both sexes look identical but 'Sadie' seems to fit. Small as she is, she is full grown, and an adult owl, having passed her juvenile years in South Dakota. Since we have had her for nearly six more years, she may even be considered middle-aged. When she is content and secure, she tends to be rounded all over, her head is a small ball, atop the larger ball of her body. However, if she feels threatened, she goes into her camouflage position and pretends that she is a broken-off snag on a tree. She straightens up tall and thin and raises her "ears" to change her profile. Her eyes close to slits and the unique coloration turns her into a broken off branch with the split clearly showing. If she sits very still, she can con her enemy into thinking so, and escape predation. When you are a very small owl, you have to be wary.

If there is anyone in South Dakota who has been wondering about what happened to a certain screech owl, she is alive and well, and living at the Northwoods Wildlife Center. She is a part of the education program at the Center, teaching visitors about owls, and their environment. You in South Dakota had the right idea. You just weren't a rehabilitation center. Of course, if you had been, as soon as he got his flight feathers, you would have released Buttons into the wild, and none of this story would have been told.

"Sorry! No touching. Patti is the smallest owl in Wisconsin. There is a smaller owl in the Southwest, but Patti wins in this area."

"What did you say she was?" asked the father.

"A saw whet owl. Her name comes from her call. All owls do not hoot. Patti sounds like a saw being sharpened on a grindstone. It's more like a cross between a buzz and a scream."

"I've heard a saw being sharpened. I can't imagine a bird sounding like that," he said.

"She has another sound, too. She sounds like a space ship!"

"A space ship?" wondered the smaller boy. "How?"

"It's a 'Beep, beep, beep' sound that seems to come from all over the woods. I have never heard it except on a recording. But it does sound like a space ship coming to visit."

"Do they live around here? Could we see one?" asked the girl eagerly.

"Yes, they do, and yes, you could. I had one in my woods one night. I got out of bed and padded out in my bathrobe and slippers to find it."

"Did you?" she asked.

"Yes. It was sitting on the limb of a pine tree. I shone my flashlight on it, and it just sat there while we both looked at each other. Then I went back to bed. But I have never heard it since."

"Maybe you scared it," offered the smaller boy.

"Maybe I did," I agreed.

There was a loud "Peep!" from the next cage.

Everyone jumped and went to see who had made the racket.

"That's Steve," I said. "He is a lesser golden plover."

"Why is he here?" asked the older boy. "He looks OK. Is he hurt?"

"Yes, he was hurt. His wing has been injured and he is not a good flyer. He would have to be good enough to fly all the way to South America to the Pampas, or at least to the southern United States for the winter. Do you know where he was found in the late fall last year?"

"No. Where?" asked the boy.

"Right over in Eagle River when he should have been flapping his way south!"

"What happened?"

"He lives up in the Arctic during the summer and had already travelled hundreds of miles. He may have bumped a window. He wouldn't be used to houses. We will never be sure. Anyway, his wing injury means he will never be released."

"What does he eat?" asked the father.

"This bird has it made. He eats meal worms, shrimp flakes, shrimp pellets and all kind of gourmet goodies. He has been adopted by one of our directors, and she brings him all kinds of plover delicacies. One of our interns also sent him a small box of shrimp flakes. Steve does very well, gastronomically speaking."

"Is this all there is?" asked the smaller boy looking at the big board door that closed the end of the trail.

"That's all there is of this trail. Now we get out into the woods." I opened the door and waited while the group walked into the enclosure.

"This is our wilderness classroom, otherwise known as 'Fort Apache'. In the summer we have scheduled programs out here. Clubs and camps sit on the wooden benches and watch a slide show. After the program, they can go upstairs where there is a picnic table and benches. The people can do a hands-on study of plants, or whatever. Mostly, they like to dissect owl pellets."

"Owl pellets?" asked the older boy.

"Remember? You watched the baby owls eat their mice. They swallowed them whole, didn't they?"

"Yes."

"Well, they digest all the good stuff. They digest all the contents of the mouse's stomach and intestines, and since the mouse is a vegetarian, the owl gets his veggies second-hand."

"Yuckhh!" exclaimed the children almost in chorus.

"That's where the owl pellets come from, though," I explained. "After all the good stuff is digested, what is left is the bones and the hair. You wouldn't want that in your stomach, would you?"

"NO!" came the response.

"What would you do about it?"

"Throw up!" replied the small boy.

"That is exactly what the owl does. He regurgitates the hair and bones in the form of a pellet. Scientists and biology teachers like to have them. If they are torn apart, it is possible to reconstruct the skeleton of the animals eaten and find out what prey the owls are eating at any time of the year. Everything is perfectly dry and it's really interesting. Most of the campers really like to see what's inside."

From their expressions, I could see that this was not the family's favorite thing. I led them through the wilderness classroom and out into the woods. The trail led past various cages and was set off by big stones all along each side.

"Somebody has been doing a lot of work," the father commented. "That's a lot of rock!"

"This is the work of our college interns. They sign up to come for the summer and work. Most are in biology, or environmental studies, or even vet students getting wildlife experience.

"They did a fine job on this path," said the father. I nodded.

"This first cage belongs to Bart, the barred owl. He is imprinted, like Ascha, the red tail you saw on the trail. Only he was imprinted by a woman in Ashland. She raised him. The DNR took him because she didn't have a license, and brought him here."

"He's got dark eyes," said the girl. "He looks very soft."

"Good for you for noticing his eyes. He is the only owl who has the dark eyes. All the rest have gold or yellow eyes. It's one way to identify a barred owl. Bart spends most of his springs and summers raising baby barred owls that are brought in. He does a fine job. He teaches them to fly and to hunt. The babies in the flight room are some that he took care of. They are about ready to be released."

"Where did the woman get him?" asked the girl.

"His nest may have been blown down in a storm. He was just found in the snow. She saved his life."

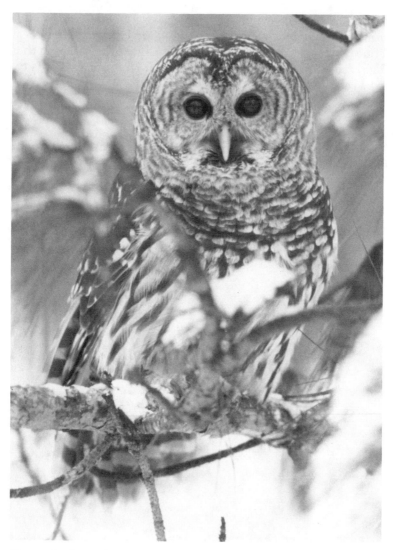

Bart, the barred owl, had to be fastened to the limb for this picture, as he is an enthusiastic flyer, not much given to sitting still for long.

BART

"I wish I could find a baby owl," the little girl said wistfully. "I'd take good care of it."

"Bart likes women better than he likes men. Probably because a woman raised him. When he goes to a program, Jacquie can pick him up easily, but he tries to bite any of the men."

"Does he go to lots of programs? Could he come to our school?" asked the older boy.

"No, because you do not live in Wisconsin. Bart cannot cross the state line. But he goes all over Wisconsin. He has even escaped twice. There is nothing wrong with his flying ability. He is not injured physically. One time at a program in a big park, he was teased by some children behind the speaker and Bart just flew away to get away from them. He was found a couple of days later sitting on a 'Handicapped Only' sign in a parking lot in the park. He was hungry and very easy to pick up and take home again."

"What was the other time?" asked the smaller boy.

Margaret looked out across the fields to the lowering sky over Lake Superior. Black clouds were rolling toward the house at an alarming speed. She glanced at the barometer and saw that it had fallen again from the mark she had set. Bad storm for sure.

Her husband and grown son came running in from the barn.

"All secure, there," Joe panted. "House OK?"

"Best I can do," Margaret answered. She looked out once more. "I hope the school knows this is coming."

"Of course they do. Don't worry. Joe watched the scudding clouds. "Lot of wind in this one!"

The mother owl was looking at the weather. The drop in barometric pressure made her feel apprehensive. Her eggs had recently hatched. She settled over her babies protectively. Her dark eyes opened and closed. It was the best she could do. The nest was an old hawk's nest which she had taken over in late February and refurbished for her family. A winter storm was always a danger, something owls had to face while nesting. Their nesting time was in the period when storm after storm rolled down from Canada. It had happened to her many times before. She turned her face to the wind. It was an excellent location for a nest. The hawk had thought so too. It was in the woodlot, but close enough to the barn to give access to a whole population of rats and mice. It was like living in a restaurant. She planned to hunt in the evening after the storm.

She waited.

The storm came closer and the winds picked up. The trees in the woodlot began to toss. Some dead branches fell. Needles of snow shot out of the storm propelled by the deadly wind. The mother owl closed her eyes and hunched down. The three babies, warm and comfortable, slept.

Then the heaviest part of the storm struck and the wind became a killer. The trees bent farther and farther, and when the gusts let up, they would snap back, and some branches would tear off. Another gust would bend the trees again. They were stressed beyond their strength. The trees themselves began to fall. The owl was clutching a branch in her nest and braced against the storm. Suddenly she felt the entire nest moving. She tightened her grip. Still the nest moved. Soon the branch she was clutching was no longer part of the nest! The nest had fallen from beneath her. She spread her wings and was lifted on the wind. The nest sailed away. The baby owlets, light as a dandelion seed, were sailing through the air at the mercy of the storm. One was lucky. It missed all the trees and sailed across an open field, landing against one of the farm buildings in a drift of snow.

"Looks like the worst part is over," Joe said as the screaming wind fell away.

Margaret looked out the window at the resulting chaos. "Look at those trees," she gasped. "We must have lost a dozen!"

"Like matchsticks," Joe agreed. "I'll go see to the barn."

"I'll help," said Jimmy. "You OK here, Mom?" Margaret nodded.

Joe shrugged into his mackinaw, mitts, and cap. He picked up a broom from the back hall as he went. The snow was dry and could be swept out of the doorway. Jimmy followed with a shovel. Joe cleared the doorway to the barn and checked his stock. All was well. He left the barn and continued his rounds to the chicken house. As he swept the snow, a movement caught his eye. There was a small moving lump in the snow at the door. Joe cleared it off with his big mitt. It turned into a small bird. He picked it up and stuffed it inside his mackinaw. Joe went back to the house.

"Guess what I have!" he teased.

"I have no idea," said Margaret. "Where's Jimmy?"

"He's clearing the snow from the path to the machine shed. Look." Joe took the baby owl out of his jacket. "A baby bird!"

"How on earth did it live through that storm? What is it?" asked Margaret looking closely at Joe's cupped hands.

"Beats me," said Joe. "With that beak, a hawk or an owl. It's too little for me to tell."

"I'd guess an owl. Look at its face."

"But it's got dark eyes. Most owls have yellow eyes."

"Let's get it warmed up and then I'll look in the book." Margaret took a berry basket out of the store room and filled it with shredded newspapers and put the baby in the midst. Then she covered the entire basket with a soft cloth. "There," she said. "Now I'll put him near the stove to stay warm. What should I feed him?"

"You look in your book," Joe grinned. "I've got some clearing to do." He put his mitts back on and went out again.

Margaret went to the bookshelf and looked up owls and hawks in her bird book. She decided that the bird was an owl of some sort, and judging by the dark eyes, probably a barred owl.

"So. You're a meat-eater are you?" she asked the owlet when she returned to the kitchen. "How about some hamburger?"

If the owl could have talked, he might have told her that hamburger was not proper baby owl food, but hamburger was what he got, and he made the best of it. Over the next few days, his diet improved as Margaret gave him ground raw chicken, and Jimmy trapped some mice in the barn.

"Look, Mom. Dinner!" he crowed, when he brought in the first mouse.

"Take that thing out of my kitchen!" howled Margaret.

"No, Mom. I'm serious. Dinner for the owl. This is what he would eat."

"Well, I'm not going to chop it up for him. He's all yours."

"I'll cut it up. You feed him. He's used to you." Jim went to the kitchen drawer for a knife.

"No!" screamed Margaret. "Not a kitchen knife! Find something else."

Jimmy looked at her for a long moment. "I'll get my old scout knife," he said.

When the mouse was suitably dismembered, Margaret gingerly picked up the pieces and fed the baby. He gulped the mouse hungrily.

"Hey. He really likes that," Jimmy said. "I'd better reset the

198

traps. Maybe we'll get him another.

Margaret overcame her aversion to cutting up mice from sheer necessity after Jimmy's spring break was over, and he had to go back to college. She had to cut the mice herself, or the owl would go hungry. By this time, she loved him dearly and he apparently felt a great affinity for her. A small fuzz-ball, he followed her around the kitchen. She set him on the counter as she prepared his dinner, and he watched intently. One day she was interrupted by the telephone, and when she came back the mouse had disappeared. She moved several things around on the counter looking. No mouse. Joe came into the house, brushing the snow from his boots and shoulders.

"What's up?" he asked as she looked around on the floor.

"I lost the mouse," said Margaret. "The phone rang and when I came back, it was gone."

"Did you take it to the phone with you?"

"No, Idiot! I wouldn't voluntarily take that mouse anywhere!"

"Maybe he ate it."

"But I hadn't even cut it in half. The whole mouse was just lying there."

"Margaret," Joe smiled, "an owl eats his mouse whole. You don't think anyone cuts up the mice for his mother, do you?"

"I didn't think about it at all," Margaret sighed. "Do you suppose that I can at last stop chopping up mice?"

"Looks that way. The baby is growing up." Joe gave her a quick squeeze and sat down to take off his boots.

After that, feeding the owl was easy. Hold the mouse by the tail and let the baby swallow it in several gulps. It was amazing how wide that little mouth could open!

The owl grew. His fuzz was replaced by handsome feathers. He was definitely a barred owl. He flew around the house and yard, but spent most of his time with Margaret. There was no question that he was her owl.

Word got around that Margaret had an owl, and people came to see him. The owl was calm and friendly. He didn't mind people at all.

Then the blow fell.

A man came to the door. "I understand that you have an owl?" he questioned.

"Yes," said Margaret. "A barred owl."

"My name is Scott McKelvey. I'm with the United States Fish and Wildlife Service." He produced his credentials. "May I see your owl?"

"Of course. Come in." Margaret stepped back from the door.

As the young man entered a dark shadow crossed the room silently, and suddenly there was an owl on Margaret's shoulder.

The young man smiled. "He seems healthy. What have you been feeding him?"

"Mice," said Margaret proudly. "He likes them best."

"You seem pretty fond of him," said Scott McKelvey. "Are you aware that it is against the law to keep a captive bird of prey?"

"It is?" said Margaret in a small voice.

"Our records don't show that you have a permit. I'm sorry, but I shall have to take him away."

"No!" pleaded Margaret. "He's used to me. He wouldn't know how to get along!"

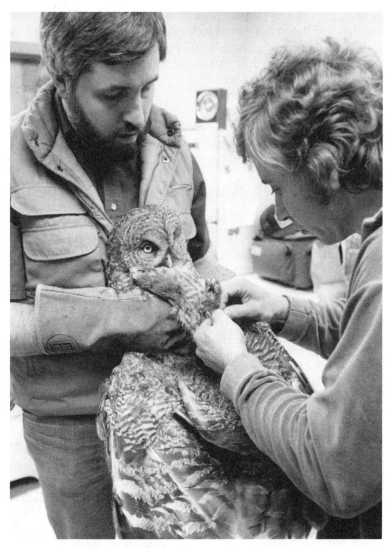

Mark holds Nanook, a male great gray owl, while Dave fixes a leg band prior to releasing the owl in a newly constructed habitat.

"That's just the problem," agreed Scott McKelvey. "He's 'imprinted'." When a baby bird looks around at about the third or fourth day to identify itself, it looks to see who is feeding it. If an owl had been feeding him, he would have known he was an owl, but what did this bird see?"

"He saw me," said Margaret softly.

"That's right. He saw you, and he imprinted on you. He doesn't know he's an owl."

"But I had to feed him. He would have died," cried Margaret. "I couldn't let him die!"

"I'm just as sorry as you are, and I know you thought you were doing the right thing. But you see, you can't let him go. He doesn't know how to get along in the wild."

"I'll take care of him. There are lots of mice in the barn."

"We can't let you do that. It's against the law. He will have to go to a licensed rehabilitation center. I'm sorry, but I have to take him." Scott McKelvey watched miserably as Margaret fought her tears. "I'm really sorry," he said again. "It's not my favorite job." He paused. "You could be fined for keeping him, but I'll write it up as extenuating circumstances. You did keep him alive." Scott paused again. "I have a carrier in the truck," he added gently. "I'll go get it." He walked back to the truck while Margaret said good-bye to her loved owl.

A week later, Bart, the barred owl, took up residence at the Northwoods Wildlife Center.

Good old Bart! Actually, he was a youngster when he came. Because he had been raised by a woman, he related better to the women at the Center than he did to the men. After several years, however, we discovered that there might be a stronger bond. Bart laid an egg! We all cheered and tried to decide what to call him now, er...her now.

"How about 'Barbie?'" I asked. "It's close enough and we could get used to it."

"Okay. Barbie. From now on Bart is Barbie," Tony decreed, and so it was written in our newsletter.

But people are hard to change. They resist. The familiar is precious. We all tried, and finally gave up. Barbie reverted to Bart, and that's what she is today.

"That was right here at the Center. One of our interns had a group program and she was showing Bart to everyone in the parking lot. She had a big glove on and thought she had Bart's jesses secure. She was wrong, and Bart slipped away and flew to a tall pine tree."

"How did you get him back this time?" asked the older boy.

"Tony went out with a mouse and held it where Bart could see it. Bart's tummy brought him home that time. When he got close, Tony reached up and grabbed his feet. You always have to control the feet of a bird of prey. If you don't he will "foot" you and that can be painful. Those talons are strong and sharp. You have to grab his feet before he can grab you."

"I'm glad he's home," said the smaller boy. "I like Bart."

"Me too." I agreed. "Now, if you will follow the trail to the very end, you will come to the great gray owls. They are the largest in North America. Just follow the trail. Keep to the left at the fork."

The family walked on through the woods.

The father looked up. "That's some cage! Who did your building?"

"Mostly volunteers. I was not here at the time, but I understand it was a tremendous job. It has space for two breeding pairs. Areas can be closed off, or the entire cage can be available as it is now. It was designed by Kay McKeever, Canada's 'Owl Lady'. She is the one who sent us the owls. They were supposed to be a

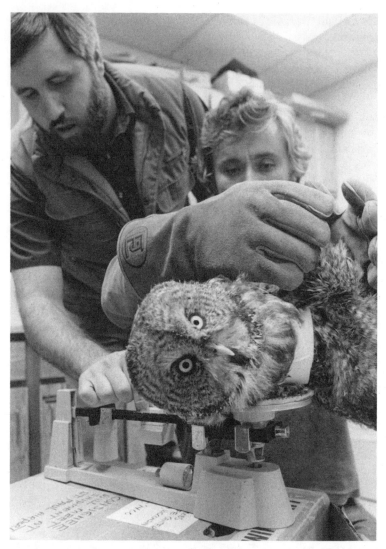

Mark and Dave weigh Nanooki, a female great gray owl, upon her arrival at the Northwoods Wildlife Center.

breeding project, but the owls thought otherwise! Can you see them?"

We had all reached the end of the trail. The owls usually sat in the far corridor of the habitat, facing the path.

"Yes, there they are. See the one up on the perch? The other is right down here on this lower perch. See him?" The mother was pointing them out.

"Wow! They are big!" exclaimed the older boy. "What do they weigh? Twenty pounds?"

"No, about five or six. They are all feathers. Their skeleton is smaller than that of the great horned owl, but their bulk is larger because of the way the feathers grow. You can stick your finger through the feathers on the top of their heads and your finger will be completely covered before you can touch scalp."

"I wouldn't want to try. They are too big."

"They are about two feet tall with a five to six foot wing span. And they can fly silently like ghost birds in the woods."

"They are beautiful, though. Very appealing," the mother said. "I like their faces."

"I do, too," I said.

"Now, follow me and we'll go and see our only educational mammals so far. These are pine martens."

We walked toward the marten cage to the right of the great grays. Skippy, our elderly gentleman pine marten, watched our approach from his corner behind his denhouse. I stopped the family.

"There. In the corner. Do you see him?"

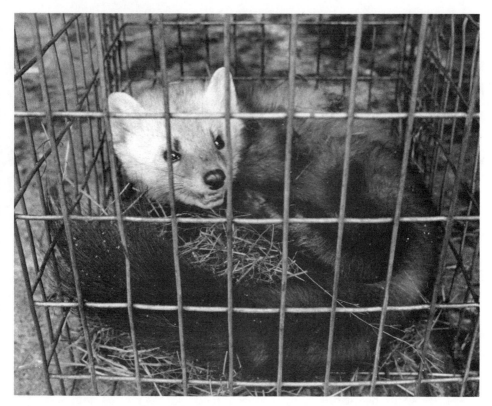

A pine marten arrives from Colorado to participate in a captive breeding program.

SAGA OF THE PINE MARTENS

Annamarie was a small person with long straight hair that reached below her tiny waist. Wide eyes and a wide smile and a sprinkle of freckles across her nose made her look like somebody's little sister. But she was Dr. Annamarie Beckel, with a Ph.D. to prove it. She was an expert on Mustelids and had done a study on the behavior of otters. She wanted to conduct a similar behavioral study on pine martens. Unfortunately, there weren't any in Wisconsin. Their habitat had been wiped out. The martens themselves had been trapped for their soft, brown fur, similar to mink. In the early part of the century, women carried huge marten muffs, had marten collars on their coats, or wore a marten capelet around their shoulders. The last known pine marten in Wisconsin was trapped in 1925. Civilization had wiped them out.

As it happened, a similar fate had overtaken the river otter in Colorado. The Wisconsin Department of Natural Resources had an agreement with the same department in Colorado to exchange Wisconsin river otters for Colorado pine martens. Already the exchange had begun, and Wisconsin river otters were cavorting in Colorado, and some Colorado pine martens were chasing around in the regrown pine forests of Wisconsin.

Dr. Beckel wanted the Northwoods Wildlife Center to initiate a captive breeding project for the pine martens, which she would oversee, and she would be able to study the behavior of the young. Mark was delighted with the idea, and the two of them began to apply for grants from foundations to fund the project. I helped. We typed. We copied. We made charts. We drew up financial estimates. We gathered the entire mess together and turned out some twenty proposals to be sent out.

Meanwhile, Mark, Dave and little Annamarie began to build a cage to hold the wily pine martens. As escape artists, they are awesome. Wire mesh in, around, and under everything was an absolute necessity! Each section of mesh had to be securely joined to every other section with pig rings. This is where Annamarie shone. For days she was out with a clamp and a bag of pig rings fastening the mesh together tightly.

Meanwhile we watched the mail for responses to our proposal. As with any nonprofit organization, money was always a problem. Finally, Mark returned from the mail box triumphant.

"We've got it! It came! Look! The Johnson Wax Foundation will fund our pine martens!" He rushed into his office to call Annamarie. Dave came in from the back room and we all read the wonderful, unbelievable letter, and sent out for a pizza to celebrate.

When the cages were finished, it was time to ask for the animals. The DNR had agreed to provide them, but it wasn't all that easy. Colorado was live-trapping them, and that was the year that blizzards hit the state, day after day, way ahead of season. The rangers were reluctant to set the traps if they couldn't be sure of being able to get to them to pick up the animals. The animals would be unharmed in the live-traps, but would die of exposure in the cold, or of suffocation if covered with deep snow. The rangers halted the trapping for that year. Several pine martens had been sent to Wisconsin, but they were young, and not breeding stock. They were released in the Nicolet National Forest to grow up a bit and propagate in the wild. We did get Skippy, though. Skippy was lucky to land in Wisconsin. In the wild, he could not have survived for another year. He was getting up in years and losing his teeth. A marten without a full set of sharp teeth wouldn't last very long. Skippy, however, suddenly had it made. He didn't have to hunt. He didn't have to kill. All he needed to do was exhibit his charming attributes to a lady marten, and food, shelter, and safety were his. He adapted quickly to his life of ease at the Wildlife Center.

I suppose this is the time to confess something which has been a deep dark secret for six years. We did get two other martens: a male and a female. They were just the right age, and we were thrilled with them. We released them from their carriers into the cage. They began exploring their new home, found the nest boxes, and if not blissfully happy in their captive situation, at least they seemed resigned to cage living.

This is what we never told anyone: The next day they were gone.

Dave came running in holding a bag of mice in his hand. "They are gone! There is no way they could get out, but they are gone!"

"They can't be!" Mark grabbed a jacket and ran out with Dave to the Marten cages. Skippy was there in his half of the cage, but the breeding pair had vanished.

"Where? How? They couldn't get out!" Mark was unbelieving.

He unlocked the padlock and opened the cage door. A thorough examination of the inside of the nest boxes proved that nobody was home. Leaves had accumulated on the cage floor. With their hands Mark and Dave examined every inch. Finally, in a corner, they found the evidence. A small hole down into the ground. They enlarged it and found where the martens had managed to tear the wire mesh away from the wood frame and squeeze out. If you were to measure a marten against the size of the hole, you wouldn't have believed it, but they did it. They were gone. Afterwards, when we could joke about it, we called it the first release of the project. At least it was a breeding pair, and somewhere around the Wildlife Center today must be a large family of pine martens all descended from the escapees.

At the time the reaction was, "How can we tell Annamarie?" She took it very well, and the following fall, we got four more martens to participate in the project. You had better be sure we mended the cage and reinforced it with oversize staples!

A pine marten is probably the most appealing of all animals to look at. He is bigger than a mink, but smaller than a fisher. He has big eyes and round perky ears and looks like something you would want to hold on your lap and pet. You couldn't be more wrong. He is a feisty, ferocious little predator, and nothing you want to put a finger near if you value that finger.

Once the pine martens were caged, they were left absolutely alone except for care and feeding. Annamarie's observation post was behind a blind, and aside from Annamarie and the caretaker, no one was permitted in the marten area.

Now we waited.

Pine martens mate in the middle of August, but the fertilized eggs do not develop until late winter and early spring. It is called delayed implantation. Any time during that period, if the female is disturbed or frightened, she can reabsorb the fertilized eggs and good-bye baby martens for that season. Since we got them in the fall of '83, and since being trapped is a harrowing situation, we knew better than to expect any young in the spring of '84.

In August of '84 Annamarie reported that they had exhibited mating play and that possibly they had mated and the female was at last pregnant. Having wished so hard for babies, Annamarie herself became pregnant, and the following spring, instead of watching marten infants, she had one of her own to care for. However, since the martens again did not produce, her absence didn't cause a problem.

We had high hopes for 1986. Again, the martens had been amorous in August, and we had acquired a mate for Skippy, who was not averse to doing his bit. We had two chances at young martens. Spring came. Nothing.

By this time, Mark had left us and had gone back to working for the airlines. He and Jill moved to LaCrosse. Bill Bauer was the new director, and he made much of the pine marten project. He was trained in research and again observed mating behavior in August, although no one had ever witnessed the actual copulation.

Surely, after five years, the martens would have young in 1987. They did not. As a breeding project, it was a bust. As a research project on the observation of behavior of the young, it was also a bust. It was very embarrassing to report year after year to the

Johnson Wax Foundation that once again the martens had failed to give birth. All heads were put together to brainstorm the reason. The only possibility we could come up with was that possibly without our knowing it, snowmobiles in winter and ATV's in summer were coming too close and the noise upset them. All our land was posted, but we had on occasion seen tracks. We put up heavy barricades to discourage trespass and put all our hopes on the next spring.

All things come to him who waits.....

The animal volunteer came tearing out of the woods and into the back door. "I heard something!" she gasped. "In the marten cage. Just little squeaks. Hurry!"

Tony, now the interim manager between Bill and Warren, jumped up and tore out the door. As he approached the marten cage he slowed down and walked quietly closer and closer. Sure enough, there were little squeaks, and the female was nowhere to be seen. The male had long ago been removed from the cage as he would be likely to eat his offspring for dinner. (I told you they were ferocious.)

"She took the mice," Janis whispered. "I fed her before I ran back. The mice are gone."

"Let's get out of here," Tony whispered back. "We don't want her upset." The two of them backed off and turned toward the Center. "From now on, the marten cage is off limits to everyone. I'll feed them myself. If anything happens, it will be my fault." He was concerned because martens are like mink, and until they are a certain age, the mother will eat her young if she feels they are endangered to save them from a possibly worse fate. For the first few weeks, the baby martens were leading precarious lives. In the cage they were safe from predators, but not from their nervous mother.

In time, Tony reported that there were two babies, which was not unusual for a first litter. They grew. They came out of the nest box and played. They climbed over the nest box and up the cage mesh. Then one day, there was only one baby. Evidence accused its mother. Something must have disturbed her. Tony went into the cage and rescued the remaining kit. The basic cage had been constructed so that portions could be closed off for just such segregation. The father was allowed back with the mother, and the baby was safely alone. He thrived.

Then we had another brainstorming session on the basic purpose of the project. The absence of any serious researcher (since Annamarie was busy observing the behavior of human young), plus the fact that the Department of Natural Resources would have liked very much to have our females in the wild, argued for termination of the project. They had received many males for release, but very few females. We decided to go that way, and called the ranger station. The Great Release was set for the following Thursday. Bob Baldwin was asked to take pictures, and when the big day came, four men from the DNR walked in the door with carrying boxes for the four martens we were planning to release. Three were females, and one was a male. We would keep old Skippy and the remaining baby. I hung around eagerly. The pine martens had been so carefully cared for that no one was permitted to go near them except the animal care people. I was not one of them. In all the time we had had pine martens, I had seen only pictures and posters. I had never seen the real, live animals. It was not long before all four had been captured and the parade of DNR men and our crews came back through the front door. The small soft animals were snarling and trying to bite through the carrying cages. We need have no fear that they had become accustomed to man. They were WILD, wild animals and ready to take up their life in the wilderness. The entire entourage went out the door and into the trucks. Bob Baldwin went with them for pictures. The Colorado pine martens became residents of Chequamegon National Forest where the second growth pines were tall and strong and just waiting for the return of the pine martens.

Jiff chose this moment to stick his nose out of his den-house.

"Look! There he is!" said the girl. "He has an orange throat!"

"Right! They have the bright orange throat and chest marking. The rest is brown. Look, he is going to show off for you."

The children watched, fascinated, as Jiff performed his gymnastics up and down the sides of the wire cage, chased his tail, jumped on and off his house and was generally delightful.

"Would they make a good pet?" asked the girl.

"No wild animal makes a good pet, these least of all. Soft and cuddly as they look, they are fierce predators and very quick to use their sharp teeth. When they have to be handled, Dave puts on heavy gloves and is the only person here who will touch them. Even old Skippy is a biter."

"I'd better just keep my cat," said the girl.

"Good idea," I answered. "But remember, he is a predator, too. If you want to be good to the wild animals, you will keep your cat inside."

"Oh, I do. He's an inside cat. He sleeps on my bed at night. He doesn't go out."

"Mine, too," I said. "All four of them!"

We walked toward the next cage.

"This is our last permanent resident. Her name is Hortense and she is a turkey vulture."

"She's ugly!" exclaimed the smaller boy.

"Don't let her hear you. You'll hurt her feelings." The smaller boy stared at me. I smiled. "She thinks she's beautiful. Watch."

"Hi, Hortense! Come over here. Come on, Sweetie. Good Bird!"

The family watched as Hortense left her far corner and began to pick her way across her cage to our side. She would take a few steps, look, tilt her head, take a few more steps, until finally she was even with us.

"Good bird! Very good! Now show us your pretty wing. Show us your wing!"

Hortense raised her one remaining wing, showing its lovely white underside and walked across the front of her cage with that wing extended.

"Good bird!" I clapped my hands. "Quick tell her how wonderful she is."

The family clapped and exclaimed over her. Hortense obliged by extending her wing again.

"Does she always do that? asked the girl in wonder.

"No, just when she feels like it. But it isn't her only trick. She also unties shoes one lace at a time. She picks the papers out of the waste baskets, and once when she was displeased with one of the volunteers, she pulled the woman's coat onto the floor and walked all over it. She has quite a personality."

"Do you let her out?"

"Yes, in the winter when she is inside. We let her walk around the Center while her cage is being cleaned. Do you see how she only has a butch cut on her head instead of being fully feathered?"

"Yes, and it's red, too," said the smaller boy.

That is one thing that keeps her clean. She eats carrion (that's anything dead) and sometimes it can be pretty rotten. If she had a fine head of feathers they would be filthy and smelly all the time, but with her butch cut, she has only to shake her head to be cleaned up again. There is nothing for rotten meat to stick to. Look at her nose. There is a hole right through it. If she gets rotten meat in her nose, she can just shake that, too, and it all flies out. Nature takes good care of its own. Each animal is made to be just right for what it does.

"What happened to her other wing?" the older boy asked.

"I don't know. She is a transfer from another rehabilitation center that discontinued its education program and transferred some of its birds and mammals to other centers. We got Hortense."

"Maybe she's not so bad," admitted the younger boy.

"She kind of grows on you," I answered. "Well, that's the end of the trail. You have seen everybody, and now we go back again."

We went through the wilderness classroom and the children all said good-bye to each resident as we went through. At the end, I locked the trail and invited them in to watch a slide show on the Center.

As the slide show ended and they stood up to go, I gave each of the children a brochure to take home, while the father, bless his heart, deposited money in our donation "dome".

And that is a tour of the Northwoods Wildlife Center. You are all invited.

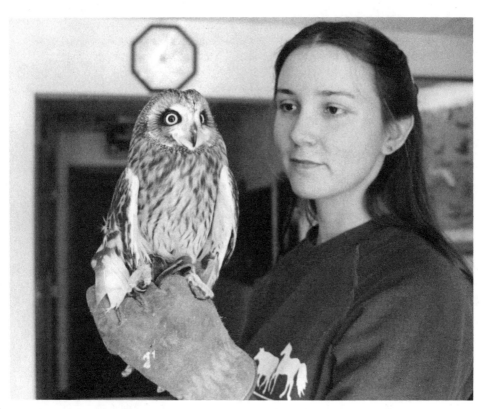

Jacquie shows off George, a short-eared owl.

APPENDIX:
THE
CENTER'S HUMANS

WILDLIFE HOSPITAL

When the Center opened in 1982, Rory Foster knew he couldn't be two places at once. The board of directors hired Mark Blackbourn to be the executive director and run the Center. Mark was a huge bear of a man with dark hair and a dark beard, and friendly eyes that twinkled when he smiled. He smiled a lot. He was an expert at rehabilitation, having done it from boyhood on the family farm. After college, however, he went to work for the airlines, married Jill, a registered nurse, and they were busy taking care of their children instead of animals, until Mark was in an accident. He was badly injured and for a period of time was hospitalized while the surgeons put him back together again. His jaw was rebuilt, and he had to wait while nature healed his damaged memory. He was given an artificial knee and had to learn to walk with it.

During this period he heard about the wildlife hospital being started in Minocqua, and he offered to serve on the board. The experience he had had as a rehabilitator turned him into the director. When I met him, he was about two months into his new job.

Mark had put an ad in the paper for volunteers to work at the Center. I answered the ad and arrived at the Center for an interview. The place was alive with volunteers already. Some were painting. Some were laying tile. Some were washing windows, and others were carrying whatever to wherever in preparation for opening the new facility. I loved Mark on the spot. He has a charisma that attracts loyalty and dedication, but with a humble, boyish quality that is endearing.

Mark asked me to wait until the Center was ready to operate, and said he really needed someone at the front desk to do office work. I was disappointed. I wanted to work with the animals. I wanted to feed the babies, help heal the injured, and be an animal Florence Nightingale. So much for dreams.

The front desk sounded dull and uninteresting. How wrong I was! The front desk was where EVERYTHING happened!

As the first summer's shake-down continued, a definite line of demarcation emerged between the front desk and the back room. The back room was all animal. The front desk was all business. Letters, mailing, reports, bookkeeping, memberships, renewals, preparing bills for payment, etc., all revolved around the front desk. Some volunteers who wanted to work with the animals left the front desk as openings came up in the back room. I filled the gaps myself, as it gave me more time to pull things together.

Mark was a PR man par excellence. His skill seemed a part of him. The Wildlife Hospital was in the papers, on television, and all over the state in Mark's programs. Insofar as public relations goes, he was able to mend fences with the Department of Natural Resources which had been Rory Foster's bête noir. Rory's dedication to the care of wild animals brooked no opposition, and no interference. His was a singleness of purpose which blinded him to the fact that some people might not agree with him, and that their reasons might be legitimate. He also tended to be very outspoken. In so doing he alienated some local persons as his idea of a wildlife hospital grew to a reality. Mark smoothed ruffled feathers. Not ALL ruffled feathers, but he did his best.

One day that fall when I was at the front desk, a young man walked in. He had blond curly hair, wide cheekbones, and a wide smile. He walked with a slight limp.

"May I help you?" I asked, thinking he might want a tour.

"I understand you are looking for volunteers," the young man answered. "I'm good with animals. I thought maybe I could help."

"We really have a lot of animal volunteers. Let me call Mark. You should talk to him." I went into Mark's office and asked him to talk to the man.

"Be right there," said Mark, who was working on the report to the board of directors.

I went back to the young man and ask him to fill out our volunteer application.

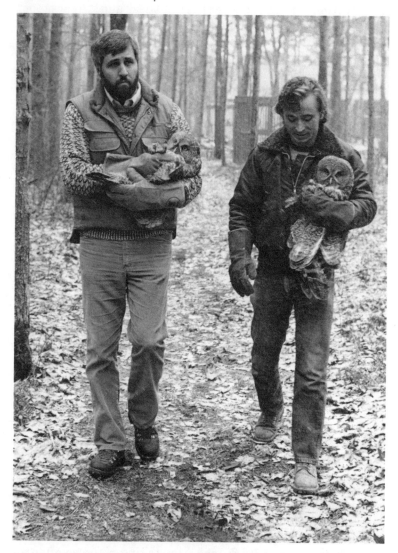

Mark and Dave carry the two great gray owls to their new habitat.

"I'm a Vietnam vet," he said. "Disabled. I can't hold a regular job, but I'd like to work with the animals." He had difficulty with his writing. His fingers did not do what he wanted them to. Obviously, muscles had been damaged. He printed the information on the blanks and finished just as Mark came out of his office.

"Hi! I'm Mark Blackbourn," said Mark, holding out his hand.

"Dave DeBauche," replied Dave, pronouncing it "DeBush."

The two shook hands and thus started the long relationship of Dave DeBauche and the Wildlife Center, which is still flourishing today.

Dave started as a volunteer, just like everyone else. But Dave came in every day. He worked with the birds and mammals. He read books. He went to rehabilitation conferences and seminars, and it wasn't long before Dave was himself a licensed rehabilitator and was working as Mark's assistant. True, there were days when he was hurting and didn't stay long. Also, he could not sit or stand for long periods of time, but had to keep changing position. But for someone to whom the doctors had said "You will never walk again," he was doing just fine. As a volunteer, he could come and go as his feeling dictated, but he gave us as much time as he could.

In March, 1985, when Mark left to go back to the airlines, Dave was considered to be the Center's rehabilitator. Bill, a former faculty member at Penn State University, who followed Mark as director, was primarily a researcher. He had obtained his Master of Science degree after completing research on the foraging preferences of white-tailed deer. His research project at Pennsylvania State University involved reintroducing injured or orphaned black bear cubs into the wild. He was also a game manager in a 13,000-acre forest preserve. At the Center he worked a little with the animals, but he was more into reading and research and spent a lot of time in his office with books and figures analyzing the Center's past performance and planning for its future. At that time Tony was doing the programs and public relations work.

Tony was a graduate of the University of Wisconsin and a Madison native. When he started as a volunteer, he was caretaking a lodge in Boulder Junction for the owners, and they didn't mind what he did with his time so long as their lodge was properly maintained. He was tall and dark and slender with a brilliant mind, deep into preserving the environment and educating the public about nature and its wildlife. He did a splendid job at it, and also learned to work with the animals. When Bill left, Tony became the manager of the Center until a new executive director could be chosen. When Warren came, Tony left. He was going back to school to get his Master's degree.

The present director is Warren Burns. He is a synthesis of all those before him, plus something extra of his own. He has Mark's charisma and appeal. He has a fine mind, and the business background that Mark lacked. He is excellent in public relations and publicity, and has carried the message of the Center all over the state and into other states besides. He has tightened up the management of the Center, and it seems that everything which has gone before was prologue to what he is doing now. If anyone can guide the Center to its goals, Warren can. Watch.

We are overseen by a board of directors which meets every other month. Committees of that board guide it and present their recommendations to the full board. It changes from time to time as board members come and go and adjustments are made to new situations.

After the first summer, Rory Foster was in Minocqua only intermittently. He sometimes filled in at the Foster-Smith Animal Hospital when Marty or T.J. Dunn had a day off. Mostly, the vet who cared for our animals was Dr. Marty Smith, Rory's partner, whom you heard about in *Dr. Wildlife,* and *I Never Met an Animal.* He was tall, with reddish blond hair. Marty was top man in his class at the vet school at the University of Iowa. He has a quick mind and a quick wit, and a dark sense of humor. He has sewn many of our patients back together again, and pulled some through that looked hopeless upon first examination. He is a serious veterinarian and a good one. He is also a very good

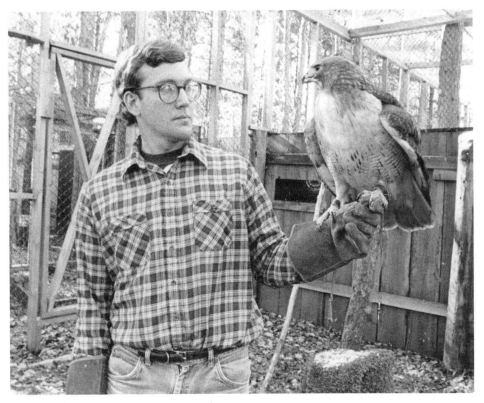

Tony Schwarz works with Ascha, the red-tailed hawk.

businessman. He and Rory started and leased out a number of veterinary hospitals in the northwoods. They also started and operated the Foster and Smith Veterinary Supply business. When Rory got sick he wanted to get his affairs in order for Linda. He sold his share of all the businesses to Marty and to his brother, Race Foster, also a vet. Marty and Race took on as a partner David Theuerkauf, who also serves on the Center's board of directors.

David Theuerkauf is a big football player-size man, married last year to a longtime friend, and daddy to a small Theuerkauf. He graduated from Michigan State University School of Veterinary Medicine. He practiced in Michigan before joining the Foster-Smith Animal Hospital in 1986. He is now one of the owners. Although he was relatively new to wildlife work when he arrived, he is now an old-timer and does excellent work.

The third member of the vet crew is Race Foster, Rory's younger brother. He was well-known to the Center personnel from when he spent his summers as a vet student working with Rory while he was going to vet school at Michigan State. He is now one of the owners both of the hospital corporation and of the mail order business. He lives in Rhinelander with his wife and children.

The newest member of the Wildlife Center team is Jacqueline Quesnell, our full-time rehabilitator. A classic beauty with high cheekbones and waist-length, black hair, Jacquie received her undergraduate degree in biology from the College of St. Theresa in Winona, Minnesota. She comes to us, however, from two years at the University of Wisconsin School of Veterinary Medicine in Madison. She had been an intern at the Center for two summers and had been so caring and compassionate, and so good at rehabilitation that we were willing to wait until she graduated so that we could have her permanently. Then, when Dave felt he needed time off from volunteering, it became more important to have someone at the Center full-time with the animals. Jacquie was approached, and after much soul-searching, agreed to come. Rehabilitation was the work she wanted, and here was a ready-made job.

Those are the Center's staff and veterinarians. We are assisted by a corps of dedicated volunteers, too numerous over the years to mention individually.

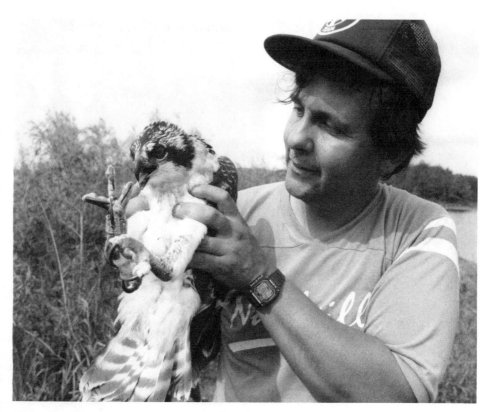

Photographer Bob Baldwin with a juvenile osprey.

Author's Biography
Sybil Ferguson

A native of the Midwest, Sybil Ferguson received her Bachelor's degree in Speech from Northwestern University in her hometown of Evanston, IL, and went on to graduate studies there, where she ultimately earned her Master's degree in Interpretation.

Her education and employment history took her to locations such as Scottsdale, AZ, Wichita, KS and Aurora, NY, but she seemed destined to return to the Midwest. After holding several challenging teaching positions from elementary and secondary education through university level instruction, Sybil branched out into business ventures and volunteer work, which led to her current position as secretary of the Northwoods Wildlife Center.

After two years as a volunteer administrative assistant there, she joined the full-time Center staff. Having worked with Dr. Rory Foster, founder of the Center and author of two other volumes about his work there, Sybil has continued working toward the goals he established for the Center.

At the time of Dr. Foster's early and tragic death from Lou Gehrig's disease in 1987, his two books, **Dr. Wildlife** *and* **I Never Met An Animal I Didn't Like** *were very successful, with wide readerships. Sybil felt the need to bring these readers up to date on the progress of the Center and to introduce the Center to new readers with her book,* **Wildlife Hospital.**

Ms. Ferguson now lives on ten acres of land in Wisconsin's Northwoods with her dog and four cats, all rescued strays. Looking forward to her 73rd birthday, she shares her acres with her wild neighbors including deer, rabbits, raccoons and porcupines.

WILDLIFE HOSPITAL

Photographer's Biography
Robert W. Baldwin

Robert (Bob) Baldwin has been the Northwoods Wildlife Center's photographer since 1983. He is best known for his loon photography which as been published in books, calendars, address books, post cards, puzzles, gift bags, etc. He has been a professional photographer since graduating high school, while taking the Associate degree program in photography at Milwaukee Area Technical College.

Baldwin is also co-owner of the St. Germain Motel & Resort in St. Germain, Wisconsin. After moving to St. Germain in June of 1982, he started his own photography business which lead him into the wildlife area. He has also produced wildlife and nature audio tapes under the NorthSound name published by NorthWord Press, Inc.

Bob lives in St. Germain, WI with his wife Jackie and sons Josh and Mike.

Also From NORTHWORD
PRESS, INC.

AUTUMN LEAVES
Ron Lanner and Bob Baldwin

If you're serious about autumn, you'll fall for Autumn Leaves, a comprehensive guide to color for the Midwestern, New England and Mid-Atlantic states. You can become the local expert on leaf color. Contains 132 splendid color photos, detailed information on the natural history of 70 species of trees, fall color hotline phone numbers for 25 states and provinces.

Softbound / 6 x 9 / 192 pages / $19.50

WHITE WOLF
Jim Brandenburg

The rare and powerful Arctic wolf is showcased in our most celebrated and beautiful book. Winner of 1989's prestigious Chicago Book Clinic Award for illustrated books, it has been hailed by Outdoor Photographer as "a landmark in nature publishing." Eloquently written, elegantly designed, it is the documentary of the author's months photographing and studying the Arctic wolves on Ellesmere Island.

Hardbound / 12-1/2 x 9-1/2 / 160 pages / $40.00
Softbound / 12-1/2 x 9-1/2 / 160 pages / $19.95

LOON MAGIC
Tom Klein

The book that launched NorthWord Press, Inc., this flagship edition continues to be the loon lover's bible. It remains, after several updates and five printings, the definitive work on the symbol of northern wilderness, the loon. The latest edition features 40 new photos, most in full-page reproductions.

Hardbound / 12 x 9-1/2 / 176 pages / $50.00
Softbound / 12 x 9-1/2 x 176 pages / $19.95

THOSE OF THE FOREST
Wallace Byron Grange and Olaus Murie

Winner of the coveted Burroughs Medal as the best book published in the field of natural history, this is a classic on forest wildlife. A celebration of the natural world, dramatized through the lives of a succession of woodland creatures and beautifully illustrated with pen and ink sketches by renowned naturalist Olaus J. Murie.

Softbound / 6 x 9 / 314 pages / $9.95

EAGLES OF NORTH AMERICA
Candace Savage

Symbol of freedom, power and integrity, the eagle is the north country's most valued summer resident. Get to know eagles through this inspiring book. Superbly researched and written text, 90 captivating photos.

Hardbound / 8-1/2 x 11 / 128 pages / $24.95
Softbound / 8-1/2 x 11 / 128 pages / $14.95

WITH THE WHALES
Jim Darling and Flip Nicklin

For the first time, a book takes you into the whales' domain under the sea. Flip Nicklin's rare and exquisite photography and accompanying text by researcher Jim Darling take you through all aspects of the whale's natural history. Covers all major species. Thoughtful and compelling.

Hardbound / 12-1/2 x 8-1/2 / 160 pages / $39.95

To receive our free color catalog or to order any of these books, call toll-free 1-800-336- 5666. NorthWord Press, Inc., P.O. Box 1360, Minocqua, WI 54548.